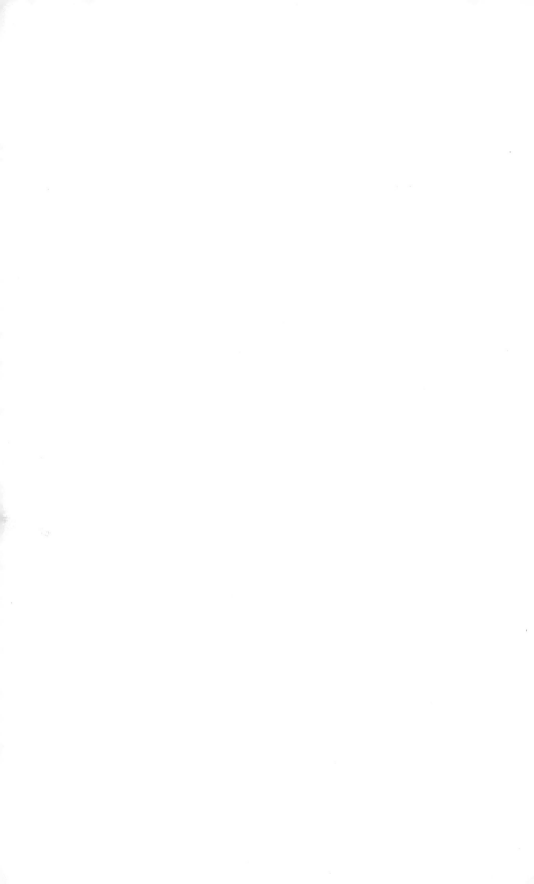

COMMISSIONING HEALTHCARE IN ENGLAND

Evidence, Policy and Practice

Edited by
Pauline Allen, Kath Checkland, Valerie Moran
and Stephen Peckham

First published in Great Britain in 2020 by

Policy Press
University of Bristol
1-9 Old Park Hill
Bristol
BS2 8BB
UK
t: +44 (0)117 954 5940
pp-info@bristol.ac.uk
www.policypress.co.uk

North America office:
Policy Press
c/o The University of Chicago Press
1427 East 60th Street
Chicago, IL 60637, USA
t: +1 773 702 7700
f: +1 773-702-9756
sales@press.uchicago.edu
www.press.uchicago.edu

British Library Cataloguing in Publication Data
A catalogue record for this book is available from the British Library

Library of Congress Cataloging-in-Publication Data
A catalog record for this book has been requested

ISBN 978-1-4473-4613-5 (paperback)
ISBN 978-1-4473-4611-1 (hardcover)
ISBN 978-1-4473-4614-2 (ePub)
ISBN 978-1-4473-4612-8 (ePdf)

Cover design by Clifford Hayes
Printed and bound in Great Britain by CMP, Poole
Policy Press uses environmentally responsible print partners

This book is dedicated to our late colleagues Dr Julia Segar

and Professor Steve Harrison, both of whom played key

roles in the development of PRUComm.

We miss them and their contributions.

Julia Segar 1959–2017

Stephen Harrison 1947–2018

Contents

List of figures and tables

Figures

Tables

List of abbreviations

ACO	Accountable Care Organisation
ACS	Accountable Care System
APMS	Alternative Providers of Medical Services
CCG	Clinical Commissioning Group
CCP	Cooperation and Competition Panel
CHS	Community Health Services
CMA	Competition and Markets Authority
CSU	Commissioning Support Unit
CQC	Care Quality Commission
CQUIN	Commissioning for Quality and Innovation
DES	Directed Enhanced Services
DH	Department of Health
DHSC	Department of Health and Social Care
DPH	Director of Public Health
DRG	Diagnosis Related Group
DsPH	Directors of Public Health
FT	Foundation Trust
FYFV	Five Year Forward View
GB	Governing Body
GMS	General Medical Services
GP	General Practitioner
HRG	Healthcare Resource Group
HSCA	Health and Social Care Act
HWB	Health and Wellbeing Board
ICP	Integrated Care Providers
ICS	Integrated Care System
JHWS	Joint Health and Wellbeing Strategy
JSNA	Joint Strategic Needs Assessment
LA	Local Authority
LES	Local Enhanced Services
LSHTM	London School of Hygiene and Tropical Medicine
LTP	Long Term Plan
MCP	Multispecialty Community Provider
MCProv	Most Capable Provider
MoU	Memorandum of Understanding
MH	Mental Health
MHS	Mental Health Services
NES	National Enhanced Services
NHS	National Health Service

NHSE	NHS England
NHSI	NHS Improvement
NICE	National Institute for Health and Care Excellence
OFT	Office of Fair Trading
OJEU	Official Journal of the European Union
ONS	Office of National Statistics
PACS	Primary and Acute Care Systems
PBC	Practice Based Commissioning
PbR	Payment-by-Results
PCCC	Primary Care Commissioning Committee
PCG	Primary Care Group
PCT	Primary Care Trust
PCR	Public Contract Regulations
PEC	Professional Executive Committee
PHE	Public Health England
PHOENIX	Public Health and Obesity in England – the New Infrastructure eXamined
PMS	Personal Medical Services
PRCC	Principles and rules for cooperation and competition
PRUComm	Policy Research Unit in Commissioning and the Healthcare System
QOF	Quality and Outcomes Framework
SHA	Strategic Health Authority
SoS	Secretary of State for Health
STP	Sustainability and Transformation Partnership
TDA	Trust Development Authority
TPP	Total Purchasing Pilots

Notes on contributors

Pauline Allen is Professor of Health Services Organisation in the Department of Health Services Research and Policy at the London School of Hygiene and Tropical Medicine and co-deputy director of PRUComm

Donna Bramwell is Research Associate in the Centre for Primary Care at the University of Manchester

Kath Checkland is Professor of Health Policy and Primary Care in the Centre for Primary Care at the University of Manchester and co-deputy director of PRUComm

Anna Coleman is Senior Research Fellow in the Centre for Primary Care at the University of Manchester

Erica Gadsby is Senior Research Fellow in the Centre for Health Services Studies at the University of Kent

Oz Gore is Lecturer in Innovation, Technology and Operations in the School of Business at the University of Leicester

Stephen Harrison was Professor of Social Policy in the Health Policy, Politics & Organisation Research Group at the University of Manchester

Imelda McDermott is Research Fellow in the Centre for Primary Care at the University of Manchester

Rosalind Miller is Research Fellow in the Department of Global Health and Development at the London School of Hygiene and Tropical Medicine

Valerie Moran is Postdoctoral Fellow in the Department of Population Health of the Luxembourg Institute of Health and a Research Associate in the Living Conditions department of the Luxembourg Institute of Socio-Economic Research

Dorota Osipovic is Research Fellow in the Department of Health Services Research and Policy at the London School of Hygiene and Tropical Medicine

Stephen Peckham is Director of the Centre for Health Services Studies (CHSS) at the University of Kent and Professor of Health Policy at CHSS and the Department of Health Services Research and Policy at the London School of Hygiene and Tropical Medicine. He is also the Director of PRUComm.

Neil Perkins was Research Associate in the Centre for Primary Care at the University of Manchester

Christina Petsoulas was Research Fellow in the Department of Health Services Research and Policy at the London School of Hygiene and Tropical Medicine

Ben Ritchie was Research Fellow in the Department of Health Services Research and Policy at the London School of Hygiene and Tropical Medicine

Marie Sanderson is Research Fellow in the Department of Health Services Research and Policy at the London School of Hygiene and Tropical Medicine

Julia Segar was Research Fellow in the Centre for Primary Care at the University of Manchester

Elizabeth Shepherd was Research Fellow in the Department of Health Services Research and Policy at the London School of Hygiene and Tropical Medicine

Lynsey Warwick-Giles is Research Associate in the Centre for Primary Care at the University of Manchester

Lorraine Williams is Research Fellow in the Department of Health Services Research and Policy at the London School of Hygiene and Tropical Medicine

Acknowledgements

This book presents independent research commissioned and funded by the National Institute for Health Research (NIHR) Policy Research Programme, conducted through the Policy Research Unit in Commissioning and the Healthcare System, 101/0001. The views expressed are those of the author(s) and not necessarily those of the NIHR, the Department of Health and Social Care or its arm's length bodies, or other government departments.

1

Introduction

Pauline Allen, Kath Checkland, Stephen Peckham,
Marie Sanderson and Valerie Moran

Introduction

The aim of this book is to bring together in one volume the most important research which the Policy Research Unit in Commissioning and the Healthcare System (PRUComm) has undertaken during the period 2011 to 2018. PRUComm is a multicentre research unit based at the London School of Hygiene and Tropical Medicine (LSHTM), the University of Manchester and the University of Kent. It is led by Professors Stephen Peckham (LSHTM and Kent), Kath Checkland (Manchester) and Pauline Allen (LSHTM). PRUComm was funded (following an open competition) by the Policy Research Programme of the English Department of Health and Social Care (DHSC) (that is, the English Ministry of Health) from 2011 onwards to provide evidence to the DHSC to inform the development of policy on commissioning and the healthcare system. The analytical work supports understanding of how commissioning operates and how it can improve services and access, increase effectiveness and respond better to patient and population needs.

Commissioning

The term 'commissioning' is used in the context of the quasi-market structures in the English National Health Service (NHS), which will be explained in detail in the following chapter. Briefly, 'commissioning' can be understood as 'the process of assessing needs, planning and prioritising, purchasing and monitoring health services, to get the best health outcomes' (NHS England, 2018a). In other words, commissioning focuses on the demand side of the NHS quasi-market (where organs of the state make decisions on behalf of patients), as opposed to the providers of care, such as hospitals. The research extends to analysing the structure and operation of the NHS healthcare system as a whole, focusing on how commissioning can be used to influence providers' behaviour. Clearly, the concept of commissioning is not confined to the English NHS. Quasi (or actual) markets were introduced into many English public services in the 1990s and the necessity for the state to undertake demand-side activities on behalf of (or in conjunction with) citizens became widespread (Le Grand and Bartlett, 1993). For example, social care has also been subject to marketisation (Forder et al, 2004). Although the term commissioning is not always used internationally, many countries have developed institutional structures for their public services in which commissioning functions are undertaken either by the state (for example, in the Italian healthcare system) (France et al, 2005) or social insurance funds (for example, in the Dutch healthcare system) (Rutten, 2004). Furthermore, it has been argued that the separation of purchasing care from its provision has an important role to play in the efficient and effective delivery of a healthcare system (Figueras et al, 2005a). Thus, although this work focuses upon the NHS in England, the findings have relevance for health systems elsewhere.

Theoretical bases of the research

Since its inception in 2011, PRUComm has undertaken an extensive range of research projects focusing on commissioning in the English NHS, including reviews of published literature, short studies to scope out issues of concern, surveys of specific NHS staff groups and a series of substantial primary research projects. The theories underlying this work are derived from several disciplines.

The research on clinically led commissioning and the structure of the public health system is underpinned by a realist evaluation approach and also draws on theories of policy implementation. Realist evaluation is a method of evaluating policies, above all, but not a universal method for researching other questions. Drawing on the work of Pawson (2013), the approach entails the elicitation of the 'programme theories' underlying policy programmes, using published documents, interviews with senior policy actors, and the views of those responsible for local implementation. Programme theories set out the expected impact of policies, using an 'if–then' logic (Weiss, 1998) and setting out why proposed policy solutions will have a beneficial effect. However, in modern policy documents programme theories are rarely clearly articulated, requiring the researcher to infer the logic. Moreover, the logic visible in published policy documents may be underpinned by additional informal logics, hence the value of interviews with senior policy actors to explore not only the ostensible purpose and intended impact of policies, but also the underlying reasoning upon which decisions are made. The value of the programme theory approach is that it allows the analyst to move beyond the question 'does this policy work?' to explore in more detail the conditions and contingencies which affect outcomes, and to explore how far both ostensible and unstated logics reflect the reality of the operation of the healthcare system. The realist evaluation approach advocated by Pawson (2013) takes this further, encouraging the researcher to define in detail the local theories underpinning approaches to policy implementation, using empirical approaches to explore and refine the *contexts* in which particular *mechanisms* lead to specific *outcomes*. These so-called 'CMO triads' provide detailed micro-level evidence about how particular policies might (or might not) work in practice, whilst at the more macro-level, analysis of ostensible and unstated programme theories reveals important avenues for investigation and provides the potential for research to inform future policy development. For example, in the study of primary care co-commissioning (see Chapter 5), interviews with senior policy makers revealed a number of aspirations underpinning the policy decision to delegate responsibility for commissioning primary care services to local Clinical Commissioning Groups (CCGs). It was found that the argument that this would support CCGs in taking a 'place-based' (a concept that pre-dates the NHS) approach to service development and delivery was undermined by the safeguards put in place to avoid conflicts of interest, in particular the establishment of a separate committee to undertake this work which was independent of the CCG governing body (GB). This finding has important policy implications, not least for current moves towards integration between primary, secondary and community services.

General practitioner (GP)-led commissioning provides a particularly fruitful topic area in which to use this approach, as the desire to increase the involvement of clinicians in commissioning services is an ideological (and rhetorical, given the considerable power and influence of the medical profession) commitment rather than an approach based upon any particular body of theory. Thus, whilst the development of the quasi-market and an approach based upon contracting for goods and services is underpinned by a sizeable body of economic and socio-legal theory (see p 9), the involvement of clinicians in planning and commissioning services relies upon a belief that clinicians will have a better understanding of patient needs and appropriate services than their managerial colleagues. This belief is not grounded in any theories of organisational or human behaviour, but rests upon an ideological commitment which owes something to the denigration of managerial work common in public discourse since the 1980s (Learmonth, 1997). In keeping with the drive to involve hospital clinicians in the management of secondary care services (Llewellyn, 2001), clinical involvement in commissioning is claimed to be an obvious 'good', without necessarily any underpinning evidence or justification. Chapter 4 explores this in more depth, reviewing the evidence relating to GP-led commissioning, and providing detailed evidence as to the conditions and contexts within which clinical knowledge may be of use in the commissioning process.

More generally, this work has drawn upon a variety of theories relevant to policy implementation, exploring the roles and impact of national policy actors such as the DHSC and NHS England (NHSE) and local policy actors such as CCGs and local authorities. In particular, the research has focused on the interaction between national and local policy makers and how national policy is interpreted and implemented at a local level. Examining policy design at a macro-level and policy implementation at meso- and micro-levels are providing a more complex, but also a more realistic, picture of the policy process. Traditional views of national policy implementation rest on theories of 'top down' implementation processes predicated on what are now more widely seen as three questionable assumptions: a chronological order in which policy intentions precede action; a linear view of the policy process underpinned by a causal link between policy intentions, policy actions and results; and a hierarchy within which policy formation is more important than policy implementation (Hupe and Hill, 2015). While the NHS is generally viewed as a centrally driven hierarchical organisation, the NHS in the UK has always been characterised by both geographical and organisational criteria and the history of the health service is one that has seen the balance between centralisation and decentralisation in a state of constant flux. The reforms of 2010 and more recent developments following the Five Year Forward View (FYFV) are in many ways just one more manifestation of the NHS continuing to wrestle with this conundrum, with repeated reorganisations motivated, in part at least, by the need to manage the tension between operational efficiency and responsiveness to local needs (assumed to be supported by local autonomy) and central control (Exworthy et al, 2010).

As the examples in the following chapters show, attempts to 'square the circles' of autonomy and control and successful implementation of national policy have adopted a number of approaches. These include the use of pilots and incentives (CCG Pathfinders, Health and Wellbeing

Boards [HWBs], Vanguards), national support programmes (Vanguards) and more latterly attempts at devolved autonomy. All of these have come with varying degrees of central stricture but, as the examples shown in this text demonstrate, local implementation is still significantly influenced by local context. However, as Checkland and colleagues (2009) concluded in their analysis of Practice Based Commissioning (PBC) 'centralized or "top-down" solutions will not work unless local context can be taken into account' (Checkland et al, 2009, page 26). What was clear in their study, and is also highlighted in the PRUComm research, is the importance of local 'sense-making' (Weick, 1979). Osborne and Radnor (2016) have argued that, for successful policy implementation, the focus needs to shift away from single public service organisations to an emphasis on the governance of inter-organisational and cross-sectional relationships and the efficacy of public service delivery systems. This is not a new idea, as it was prominent in studies of the 'Great Society' programme in the United States in the 1970s, but it is perhaps notable that the more fragmented NHS which has developed since 2000 (driven by a focus on competition and choice) has more recently spawned a range of policies designed to increase integration between organisations and sectors. Reflecting this, discussions of policy failure or the implementation gap (Pressman and Wildavsky, 1973; Gunn, 1978) have been supplemented by more complex systems thinking informed by notions of unpredictability, non-linearity and adaptability (Plsek and Greenhalgh, 2001; Best and Holmes, 2010; Pawson, 2013) and understanding national and local policy developments in the NHS requires more nuanced approaches that address concepts of localism, autonomy, accountability and intra- and inter-organisational analyses.

The economics of markets (and their opposite, hierarchies) in conjunction with more sophisticated theories of cooperation underpin the analysis of competition and cooperation in the NHS quasi-market. The core notion in the economics of markets is that there are willing and rational buyers of goods or services (demand) and willing and rational providers of goods or services (supply). In order for a market to operate efficiently, there need to be sufficient numbers of each for competition to occur. Economic theory states that, in these circumstances, the price at which goods/services are purchased will be the most efficient one (the equilibrium) (Allen, 2013). In pure markets, demand is expressed by the individuals who receive the goods/services making choices themselves and paying their own money. It is assumed that consumers are able to find and process sufficient information about the goods/services to make rational choices. These conditions ensure that each person's individual utility is maximised, as they each are the best judge of what will achieve this. Thus, the market has produced value for money by allocating resources to the best use (Allen, 2013). The mechanism by which demand and supply is brought together is a contract, under which the parties are free to agree whatever terms they wish, and which will be enforced by the legal system. In perfect markets, not only is efficiency achieved, but so is accountability, as each consumer has made their own decision based on adequate information, and the terms of the agreement between the consumer and supplier can be enforced against the supplier using contract law (Allen, 2013). Although, as will be explained in Chapter 2, the English NHS quasi-market does not exhibit all of the foregoing characteristics (in particular, patients do not pay directly for healthcare, and demand decisions are mainly made on their behalf by commissioners), the central notion that competition on the supply side is the best way to achieve efficiency and accountability for quality of care is the foundational theory for understanding the principles behind the NHS quasi-market, and the way in which commissioning is meant to operate in that market.

In addition to economic theories of markets, economic theories of hierarchies are also important when understanding how commissioning in the NHS operates in practice. In contrast to markets, where power is distributed among all participants, in a hierarchy there is a single person or group at the top with the most power and authority, and each lower level represents a lesser authority. Instead of competition between freely operating providers, decisions about supply are made inside the hierarchy using authority. Consumers do not make direct consumption decisions either: the hierarchy allocates goods and services to them. Classic economic theory sees hierarchical structures as relatively inefficient compared to markets. This is because centralised authority is employed to make decisions about the use of resources, rather than the 'invisible hand' (Smith, 1776) of the market, under which many individual decisions are aggregated to form an equilibrium. The former may reduce efficiency in production of goods/services. Furthermore, Williamson (1985) notes that the lack of strong incentives in hierarchies, compared to contractual relationships in markets, is likely to reduce the efficiency of command and control structures.

Hierarchies introduce additional questions about accountability to consumers of services which do not occur in pure markets. It is primarily decisions on the demand side which become more complex as decisions are not made by each consumer, but by someone else in the hierarchy on their behalf. In these circumstances, the notion of holding someone to account for those decisions becomes meaningful. A useful definition of accountability is 'a relationship between an actor and a forum, in which the actor has an obligation to explain and to justify his or her conduct, the forum can pose questions and pass judgement and the actor may face consequences' (Bovens, 2007, page 450). There are various ways in which these decision makers can be held to account, including (depending on the circumstances) use of legal sanctions, locally agreed contracts and public elections. All of these have their problems (Hirschman, 1970; Stewart and Ranson, 1988; Longley, 1990). As Hughes and Dingwall (1990) and later researchers (Allen, 2002b; Petsoulas et al, 2011) show, the hierarchical nature of the NHS, in which many detailed policies are made at the centre and all local organisations are required to carry these out, remains a useful way of understanding how local commissioners and providers behave in the NHS, despite the formal quasi-market structures.

The third aspect of economic theory which is important for understanding the behaviour of commissioners in the NHS quasi-market is that of cooperation. Despite the fact that the fundamental theory of markets is based on the notion of competition, there is a large amount of economic theory which explains why and how market actors choose to cooperate rather than compete, and how this cooperation can produce more efficient outcomes. Two particular theories are salient for the research reported in this book. The theory of 'co-opetition' (an interpretation of game theory from the perspective of organisational strategy) suggests that organisations can compete and cooperate simultaneously to mutual benefit (Brandenburger and Nalebuff, 1996). Brandenburger and Nalebuff (1996) suggest that rather than aiming to do better than their competitors at all times (as is assumed in conventional theories of markets) organisations would benefit from tailoring their strategies to cooperate with each other in order to increase the size of the market ('value creation') and then to compete with each other to secure their share of the improved market ('capturing value'). Whilst it is not appropriate to talk about increasing the size of the market in terms of the provision of NHS healthcare as the budget for healthcare is fixed at the point at which organisations are planning and providing services, it has been suggested that the equivalent benefits would be gained through making the existing budget work more effectively (Goddard and Mannion, 1998), through increasing innovative practice or reducing the cost of organisational interrelationships. Co-opetition theory is based on a fundamental belief that the pursuit of win/lose strategies is often counterproductive in a business environment, as tactics which result in a short-term gain at the expense of a competitor may result in a retaliatory strike, turning interactions into lose/lose outcomes. Co-opetition suggests that to be successful, organisations should be more flexible about their decisions to compete, and be more open to cooperating with competitors when it is mutually beneficial. The notion is that it is possible to combine the two approaches to mutual advantage (Bengtsson and Kock, 2000).

The second very useful theory of cooperation is derived from the seminal (and Nobel prize-winning) work of Elinor Ostrom (2005). Ostrom is concerned with common pool resource problems, specifically how to encourage cooperation between participants in situations where there is a limited common resource. It is traditionally seen that there are two possible solutions to common resource problems. Firstly to treat the common pool resource as a private good, and secondly to introduce government regulation. However, Ostrom suggests that individuals can self-organise to solve collective problems, without direct control by the government, and can establish and enforce rules limiting the appropriation of common pool resources. The framework identifies the principles, rules and characteristics which are shared by systems that successfully self-manage (Ostrom, 2010). The most common application of this framework is to situations where there is a limited physical resource to be shared, for example the framework has been used in studies of irrigation systems (Benjamin et al, 1994) and forest governance (Gibson et al, 2000). However there are some similarities between common resource problems and the allocation of the resources to support the planning and provision of services in local health economies in the English NHS. Local NHS commissioners have fixed annual budgets to be used for the provision of health services to the local population. These budgets are limited and finite. If used wisely across the health community, and if organisations coordinate their activities, then resources will go further, will be used more efficiently, and savings in one area can be spent in another. If organisations all took their individual maximum, they would not be willing to help with the development of service configurations which reduced their own incomes, although these new ways of delivering health services might be most efficient for the health community as a whole. Eventually, as a result of this, there may occur general degradation in services in the area due to the development of a commissioner deficit or because resources are not being distributed in an efficient way. Ostrom identifies a key contextual factor as being the rules governing organisations' (or individuals') behaviour.

Related to market, hierarchy and cooperative theories discussed on pages 5–8, institutional economics and socio-legal concepts underlie the approach to understanding the use of contracts in the

NHS quasi-market. Contracting for health is challenging because of the complexity of health services and concomitant high levels of asymmetric information and uncertainty between providers of care and its purchasers (Arrow, 1963). Due to the high level of expertise and specialisation in the delivery of health services, it is difficult for the purchaser to know that the agent is fulfilling the terms of the contract. Furthermore, it is also difficult for purchasers to ascertain the costs of providing care and to measure all aspects of the quality of care. It is possible that due to this 'information impactedness' (Williamson, 1975), opportunism may occur and one party may take advantage of the other's information deficit. The existence of such imperfect information means that it is particularly costly to enter into contracts, as the more imperfect the information the higher the costs of negotiating and writing contracts, and also monitoring, enforcing and renegotiating contracts. Given these circumstances, the purchaser may wish to use the mechanisms of the contract to share the financial risk with those providing services. Through using pricing and payment structures which provide financial incentives and penalties, purchasers can encourage the provider to deliver the outcomes desired by the purchaser, thus in part mitigating the problems caused by imperfect information.

Economic and socio-legal theories of contracting generally, together with empirical evidence on contracting and pricing in healthcare, indicate that the allocation of financial risk is often handled differently from the stipulations of formal contractual provisions (Williamson, 1985; Petsoulas et al, 2011). It is also the case that parties to long-term contracts often do not plan and specify their contractual relationships completely (Macaulay, 1963). In these circumstances, the relational norms of contracts might evolve to predominate, permitting efficient trade (Macneil, 1981). These relational aspects of contracts allow adjustments to be made to the initially agreed terms during the course of the contractual relationship to deal with unforeseen contingencies (Vincent-Jones, 2006). Risk can be managed by the parties as events arise (when cooperative strategies can be developed) (Sabel, 1991). In particular, financial risk, which is formally allocated through pricing mechanisms and payment structures, is likely to be dealt with by a range of methods, including post hoc adjustments to pricing, which may not be formally recorded as variations to contract.

Extensive research on contracting for healthcare, in the NHS (eg Roberts, 1993; Flynn et al, 1996; Raftery et al, 1996; Hughes et al, 1997; McHale et al, 1997; Allen, 2002b; Marini and Street, 2007; Petsoulas et al, 2011) and elsewhere (such as Ashton 1998, in respect of New Zealand, and Palmer and Mills 2005, in respect of South Africa) has shown that, indeed, contracts for healthcare tend to be based on relational norms, as well as varying degrees of 'discreteness'. All contractual relationships contain a range of both types of these norms. The former may include trust and flexibility, and may well entail changes in the terms of the contractual relationship which are at odds with the written document signed by the parties. The latter discrete norms include matters such as planning and precision. It is the balance between them which varies, depending on issues such as the complexity of services under contract.

Structure of the book

The book is structured as follows. Crucially, **Chapter 2** provides the context, setting out the organisation and governance of commissioning in the NHS. It includes a short summary of the architecture of commissioning pre-Health and Social Care Act (HSCA) 2012, and highlights the important changes which were brought about by the Act, including the abolition of Primary Care Trusts (PCTs) and Strategic Health Authorities (SHAs) , the establishment of CCGs, the creation of NHSE, transfer of commissioning responsibilities to different bodies (such as public health) and the setting up of local HWBs. The chapter also highlights the programme theories underlying the HSCA 2012, in particular the commitment to competition as a means of improving services and the expected benefits of greater clinical involvement in commissioning.

The subsequent chapters report a series of research projects which PRUComm undertook between 2011 and 2018. As only a selection of PRUComm research is covered in this book, readers should note that there are several topics in respect of commissioning healthcare which are not discussed. These include the work of Commissioning Support Units (CSUs) (which are independent organisations contracted by CCGs to carry out many commissioning and contracting functions on their behalf; see, for example, Petsoulas et al, 2014). The book does not deal with differences between England and the other home countries, where there has been less emphasis on quasi-markets (see, for example, Allen et al, 2016, concerning the changes to the commissioning system in Wales). And the commissioning of specialist healthcare services in England, such as that provided in prisons or to the armed services (see, for example, Byng et al, 2012), in respect of prison healthcare, is not covered; nor is specialist commissioning by NHSE (see, for example, Checkland et al, 2018a).

Chapters 3, 4 and 5 focus on the concept of clinically led commissioning which was brought to the fore by HSCA 2012, using realist evaluation and policy implementation approaches as a conceptual foundation. Thus, the book places more emphasis on the organisation and development of commissioning than on its effects on providers of care (although both Chapters 6 and 7 include consideration of this). **Chapter 3** deals with the development and early operation of CCGs. Building upon the context set out in Chapter 2, the factors affecting early CCG development are examined, highlighting the complexity of their governance structures, approaches taken to engaging with their members and the development of external relationships with a wide range of new bodies. An explicitly 'bottom-up' approach to policy implementation was found, with CCGs given considerable leeway in developing their structures and processes. As a result, the history of previous commissioning structures and arrangements played an important role in the development of each CCG, as did the approach taken by local leaders and by the PCT/developing NHSE local team. Engagement with local bodies such as HWBs and local authorities were also significantly affected by local history and geography. It was found that the approach taken by NHSE to CCG development, with early freedom to develop as they chose, increasingly curtailed by more prescriptive guidance and a complex assurance regime, led to some frustrations for those involved. **Chapter 4** looks at the evidence about clinical engagement in GP-led commissioning. Extending and strengthening clinical leadership was one of the key elements of the HSCA 2012. However, this idea was not new, and this chapter reviews the evidence on the role of clinicians in commissioning and how this has contributed to the delivery of healthcare services since the early 1990s. It examines the nature of clinical engagement/involvement in the various GP-led commissioning models that have been introduced into the NHS. Drawing on a review of the literature and the research on CCGs, the chapter shows how the extent of clinical engagement has varied between the various schemes. GP commissioners have historically been more successful in influencing the work done by GP practices than in making broader changes to services provided by secondary care. The chapter goes on to explore the claims made both by those involved and in official documents about how greater involvement of clinicians in CCGs – and in particular GPs – will enhance commissioning practice. This is tested against evidence from the study of CCGs, showing how the engagement and involvement of GPs requires careful attention to detail. Using a realist approach to evaluation, the contexts and mechanisms associated with successful – and unsuccessful – GP involvement in commissioning are highlighted. **Chapter 5** then reports research on the more recent policy of allowing CCGs to commission primary care services. In 2014 CCGs were invited to volunteer to take on responsibility for commissioning services from their member GP practices in addition to their wider responsibilities for commissioning acute and community services. This chapter explores the history of primary care commissioning and financing in England, and discuss the broad policy objectives which underpinned this significant change in CCGs' role and scope. These objectives include the need to move to a 'place-based' approach to commissioning, and the need for a more effective linkage between the commissioning of primary and secondary care services in order to support movement of services into the community. Over time, most CCGs have moved to take on full delegated responsibility for commissioning GP services, and have established functioning primary care commissioning committees, with little evidence of significant problems associated with conflicts of interest. The development of local additional 'quality contracts' and investment in infrastructure and premises have been important issues, with few CCGs seeking to establish larger-scale contractual changes. There have been significant local legacy issues in some areas relating to unclear contracts and poor handover of responsibilities from NHSE. The current legislation, under which statutory responsibility for commissioning primary care services remains with NHSE and is delegated rather than transferred to CCGs, presented some problems, particularly for those CCGs that wished to work together across a broader geographical footprint.

Chapters 6, 7 and 8 deal with issues related to the role of commissioners in the healthcare system. Chapters 6 and 7 focus on quasi-market issues and are underpinned by the economic theories discussed on pages 5–9. **Chapter 6** reports a longitudinal study of commissioners' (and providers') use of competition and cooperation. This chapter reports research which aimed to investigate how commissioners in local health systems managed the interplay of competition and cooperation in their local health economies, looking at acute, mental health (MH) and community health services (CHS). The understanding of the regulatory context of the NHS market by both commissioners and providers of care was unclear. There were differences between local areas in terms of the volume and mode of using competition as a commissioning mechanism, with some having more enthusiasm for and experience in running competitive procurements than others. Commissioners noted that the procurement process was very resource intensive. By 2018 there was a marked decline in the appetite to use competition, especially for large-scale service reconfigurations. Collaborative planning involving key local providers was a preferred way for CCG commissioners to approach large commissioning tasks. **Chapter 7** reports two studies of the use of contractual mechanisms in commissioning. Two of the major uses of the contract are to allocate resources to providers through pricing and to act as an instrument to improve services. This chapter reports two aspects of research on contracting in the NHS. The first investigates how the policies to use contractual mechanisms including financial risk allocation work in practice. Most of the contractual relationships between NHS-owned acute providers and commissioners were characterised by the use of general annual financial settlements outside the terms of the contract. It was not always possible for commissioners to pay the full contractually designated amount for activity undertaken, as their budgets were not always sufficient. This behaviour appeared to be increasing over time. The second study comprises a review of the evidence concerning new forms of contract being introduced into the NHS: alliance and outcome-based contracts. These are aimed at facilitating the integration of services and improving quality of care. Evidence from other sectors indicates that new models of contracting may result in cost savings, including a reduction in capital costs, the development of innovations and benefits in terms of time. But there are high transaction costs in relation to the process of contract negotiation and specification. The evidence base regarding improvements in the quality of services is not convincing. These models carry a number of potential governance issues concerning their implementation in the NHS, and are at risk of failing to satisfy public sector governance objectives, including accountability, integrity and transparency. **Chapter 8** reports research on the changing role of commissioning in the restructured public health system. The chapter discusses how public health commissioning responsibilities have changed and become more fragmented, being split amongst a range of different organisations, most of which were newly created in 2013. It focuses on discussing how the reorganisation substantially changed the way public health commissioning is done, who is doing it and what is commissioned, since the reforms. There have been significant changes in commissioning processes, with important consequences for what health improvement services are ultimately commissioned. There are also new opportunities for creativity and joining public health with wider determinants of health (such as housing and leisure).

Finally, **Chapter 9** draws together key themes arising from the book about issues raised by commissioning in the context of a quasi-market for healthcare in the English NHS, such as governance and accountability, clinical engagement, coordination and fragmentation. The chapter presents an overview of how commissioning in health and healthcare has developed since 2010 and what the implications are for the future in the light of recent developments moving away from market-style mechanisms to forms of local collaborative planning.

2

Context: commissioning in the English NHS

Imelda McDermott, Pauline Allen, Valerie Moran, Anna Coleman, Kath Checkland and Stephen Peckham

Introduction

This chapter provides a brief contextual summary, setting out the organisation and governance of commissioning in the NHS. It gives an overview of commissioning from the creation of the internal market in the late 1980s to its consolidation pre- and post-HSCA 2012, and highlights the important changes which were brought about by the HSCA 2012. The chapter highlights the programme theories underlying the internal market and the HSCA 2012, in particular the commitment to competition as a means of improving services and the expected benefits of greater clinical involvement in commissioning. The architecture of commissioning following the HSCA 2012 is outlined and an overview of developments since the Act is presented.

It is perhaps important to note here that clinical involvement in commissioning has been variously referred to as 'clinically-led' and 'GP-led'. In its earliest manifestations (GP fundholding) there was a clear policy commitment to the involvement of local GPs (primary care physicians) in commissioning. As noted in Chapter 1 this policy was driven by a belief in the value of local clinical knowledge, rather than by any evidence of its value. Over time, emphasis in policy has shifted between 'GP-led commissioning' (such as fundholding, PBC) and 'clinically led commissioning' (such as Primary Care Groups [PCGs]). The use of the wider term 'clinically led' has been used by policy makers to signal a commitment to the wider engagement of other clinicians such as nurses and hospital consultants, often in response to representations from other professional groups. Thus, in their first iteration, CCGs were explicitly intended to be GP-focused, but during a consultation period the rules were amended to mandate the involvement of both a nurse and a hospital consultant on CCG governing bodies, and policy documents reflected this by referring to 'clinically led' commissioning. However, in practice, clinically led commissioning has generally meant GP-led commissioning, with the involvement of other clinicians tokenistic at best. In this book, for consistency, the term 'GP-led commissioning' is used, but acknowledge that policy has, at times, tried to promote a wider clinical engagement beyond local GPs.

Internal market/purchaser–provider split – the origins of 'commissioning'

The NHS was established initially in 1948 as a hierarchical public organisation. In the late 1980s a quasi-market, incorporating competition between providers of care, was seen by the then Conservative government as the best form of governance structure for the NHS, which would improve value for money and quality of care (Department of Health, 1989). A quasi-market for community, secondary and tertiary healthcare was introduced by means of a split between the purchasers of care – health authorities and GP fundholders (see Table 2.1) at the time – and its providers. The providers of healthcare were constituted into publicly owned 'self-governing trusts', which were supposed to compete with each other, thereby enhancing technical efficiency (that is, ensuring the greatest output for the least resources used: 'value for money') (Department of Health, 1989). The system of annual budget allocations was to be replaced with one based on negotiated contracts between purchasers and providers.

The Conservative government's reasons for the introduction of the internal market into the NHS were made explicit in *Working for Patients* (Department of Health, 1989). First was the desire to achieve better 'value for money' (Department of Health, 1989). Proponents such as Enthoven (1985) contended that technical efficiency was more likely to be achieved in a situation of competition between providers than in a structure (such as a hierarchy) which effectively contained monopoly providers. Competition would incentivise providers to reduce costs and increase quality in order to maintain or increase its market share. A second reason was that it would stimulate staff and professionals to behave in a more responsive manner in relation to the needs and desires of patients (Department of Health, 1989), so that patients would not choose an alternative provider. A third reason was that patients should be given a greater choice of the services available

(Department of Health, 1989). This would encourage providers to improve efficiency, quality and responsiveness in order to attract more patients. The introduction of quasi-markets in the NHS was reflective of the overall trend towards marketisation of public services, extension of consumer choice and diversification of providers in the UK (eg Greener and Powell, 2009).

At the end of the 1990s the New Labour government 'went with the grain' and retained the quasi-market structures, despite also focusing on top-down, hierarchical measures, such as performance targets (Tuohy, 1999; Allen, 2002a). After the general election in 2001, there was an increased emphasis on markets and choice (Department of Health, 2007a; Hughes and Vincent-Jones, 2008; Allen, 2009b). The key measures of the New Labour policy on commissioning healthcare services were:

(i)   Demand-side reform: designed to improve services by promoting enhanced patient choice. It was thought that patients would avoid underperforming hospitals, and the prospect of losing funding under the cost-per-case Payment-by-Results (PbR) pricing system would create incentives to improve quality.

(ii) Transactional reform: a national tariff of fixed prices for procedures, known as PbR (Department of Health, 2007b). Each episode of care reimbursed (or lost to another provider) would be charged at national tariff rates.

(iii) System management and regulation: in addition to the continuing role of the hierarchical, top-down command-and-control system run from the Department of Health (DH) (and since 2013, NHSE) in the form of compulsory policies, the economic regulation of this system was undertaken by an arm's length body, the Cooperation and Competition Panel (CCP) which advised the DH in accordance with the *Principles and rules for cooperation and competition* (PRCC) (Department of Health, 2010c). The other important regulator was the independent regulator of Foundation Trusts (FTs) called Monitor (Allen, 2006).

(iv) Supply side reform: the first reform to the supply side under New Labour was the introduction of NHS FTs. While FTs were still owned by the state, they represented a more autonomous organisational form (Davies, 2004; Department of Health, 2005; Allen et al, 2012). Commissioners were also encouraged to engage with new providers from the 'third sector' (Department of Health, 2006a) and for-profit providers were also encouraged to enter the NHS quasi-market on a larger scale. (Allen and Jones, 2011)

Many scholars have noted that the competition in the market for healthcare services, and the NHS in particular, has several important limitations (Roberts, 1993; Allen, 2013). It has been shown that the English NHS operates as a quasi-market as 'it is not possible to construct a market conforming to classical economic principles in respect of healthcare' (Allen, 2013: 8). The main issues preventing full market competition from taking hold in the NHS are asymmetry of information, which limits the exercise of patient choice, the mediating role of purchasers/commissioners of healthcare on the demand side and low competition between providers and interference from government hierarchy on the supply side (Allen, 2013).

The severe limitations of competition in the quasi-market for healthcare undermine the programme theories underpinning the rollout of competition in the NHS, namely that the competition increases quality and efficiency of services. Extensive research, based on transaction costs theory (Coase, 1937; Williamson, 1985), demonstrates that markets are not always the most efficient institutional structures compared to more hierarchical forms (eg Joskow, 1987), and this research extends to health services (eg Croxson, 1999). Hierarchies may be more efficient in the provision of healthcare as market incentives may be detrimental to efficiency and quality of care where those incentives cannot be effectively harnessed for the public good. Moreover, a hierarchy allows strategic planning and allocatively efficient decisions to take place at the appropriate level of aggregation (Allen, 2013).

While the New Labour government abolished fundholding practices, the clinical element of commissioning was retained with the establishment of PCGs in 1999. PCGs brought together all GPs in a locality (see Table 2.1), along with community nurses, social services, the Health Authority and lay representatives (Audit Commission, 2000). The New Labour government declared that local doctors and nurses would drive the organisations, and GP practices were viewed as the building blocks. PCGs were established to purchase or 'commission' services for the local community. The ultimate aim was for all PCGs to develop into independent trusts comprised of GPs and nurses that would commission primary, secondary and community health services for the local population. These organisations were called PCTs and they were responsible for 80 per cent of the NHS budget. In 2000, the government announced that, in England, all

PCGs should become PCTs. PCTs would have a clinical committee, the Professional Executive Committee (PEC), chaired by a GP and a Trust Board comprising executive directors (including the PEC Chair, other clinicians and managers), lay non-executive directors and a lay chairperson (Department of Health, 2000). In 2002, Health Authorities were aggregated into SHAs which were responsible for the strategic supervision of NHS provider trusts and PCTs.

To further enhance GP involvement, in 2005 the government introduced a universal roll-out of a scheme named PCB to address the perceived lack of GP engagement in the PCT commissioning process. There was a requirement for 'universal coverage' (Department of Health, 2005), meaning that all GP practices in England were 'significantly engaged' by December 2006. PBC was officially seen as a complement to patient choice of provider, PbR and the roll-out of FTs, all leading towards a 'patient-led NHS'.

Under PBC, GP practices were provided with an 'indicative budget' with which to commission services for their patients. The scope of this budget was not fully specified by the DH, but as a minimum it included hospital activity covered by PbR (that is, hospital outpatient, inpatient and emergency care), CHS, MH and prescribing. PCTs provided the management support that practices needed to undertake PBC. Although the scheme was voluntary, the successful enrolment of practices in the scheme became a key performance indicator for PCTs. Nevertheless, the development of PBC was patchy. This was due to factors including disruption arising from the reorganisation of PCTs in 2006, a lack of prioritisation of PBC, relations between PCTs and GPs and a lack of understanding about what PBC could be used to achieve (see Checkland et al, 2008); Coleman et al, 2009). Evaluation suggested that, whilst PBC groups had limited success in catalysing widespread service redesign, there was evidence of a commitment to and progress towards the performance management of participating practices, alongside a variety of incentive schemes designed to improve access to services and the range of services available in primary care (Coleman et al, 2009).

Coalition government – HSCA 2012

A fundamental intention of the HSCA 2012 was to 'liberate professionals and providers' from top-down control. It sought to do this by placing clinicians at the heart of commissioning decisions, complemented by an emphasis upon localism to bring commissioning decisions closer to individual patients. This would achieve the necessary quality, innovation and productivity to enhance clinical and cost outcomes.

The Act established CCGs as clinically led organisations with responsibility for commissioning the majority of health services. This was intended to lead to improved outcomes because clinicians would be afforded greater autonomy to use their professional experience to make judgements about which services to commission.

Table 2.1 illustrates the various GP-led commissioning initiatives which have been introduced in the NHS from the start of the internal market to the coalition government, and sets out their scope.

Under the HSCA 2012, the key duties and responsibilities for improving health and coordinating local efforts to protect the public's health and wellbeing were transferred from the NHS to local authorities (LAs). LAs were given responsibility for commissioning public health services including sexual health, drug and alcohol and health checks. This would enable the coordination and integration of public health with relevant services delivered by LAs such as housing, the environment and transport, resulting in a greater impact on the wider determinants of health at local level.

The White Paper was couched in the language of localism and decentralisation, with an emphasis on freeing CCGs from central control, allowing them to establish themselves in ways best suited to local conditions and to work out local solutions, in partnership with LA colleagues. This new localism was intended to lead to improved outcomes because of a focus upon local needs, in which 'local' is defined as a size sufficient to operationalise contracting and to manage financial risk. In addition, the 2010 White Paper proposed to build on the power of LAs to promote wellbeing, via establishing statutory bodies called HWBs, which would provide local democratic oversight and support joint working between the NHS and LAs.

A new statutory body, the NHS Commissioning Board (known operationally as NHSE – not to be confused with the NHS Executive, 1996–2002 – was created with the intention of reducing the abilities of the Secretary of State for Health (SoS) to 'micromanage and intervene'. The SoS would provide a 'short mandate' to NHSE to oversee the provision of health services but would lose powers to intervene in relation to any specific commissioner. The establishment of NHSE as an 'arms-length' body removed political interference and control.

The mandate issued by the SoS sets out the duty of NHSE and the nature of its work. The mandate was intended to set direction

Table 2.1: GP-led commissioning since 1991

Date	Innovation	Scope of scheme
1991–95	Introduction of purchaser–provider split	Provision of care split from purchasing, with Health Authorities established as geographical organisations responsible for strategic planning and purchasing of healthcare for geographical populations
	GP fundholding	Volunteer GP practices provided with budgets to purchase care for their registered populations. Budgets covered elective care and prescribing. Savings retained by individual practices, could be invested in practice premises
	Locality commissioning and GP commissioning	A variety of locally developed models of GP involvement, with varying degrees of power and responsibility. Use of savings locally determined
1995	Total Purchasing Pilots (TPP)	An extension of GP fundholding. Volunteer groups held a budget covering a range of services which was agreed with local Health Authority. Savings reinvested in services by the group
1997	New Labour government elected – GP fundholding abolished, PCGs established	PCGs officially subcommittees of Health Authorities. Responsible for commissioning full range of services. GP majority on Board. Underspends could be reinvested, but may result in recalculation of budgets
2000	PCGs became PCTs	Health Authorities abolished, PCTs given responsibility for commissioning full range of services and providing CHS. GPs no longer in a majority, few GPs involved. Underspends could be reinvested, but may result in recalculation of budgets
2005	PBC introduced	Volunteer groups of GPs given indicative budgets covering variable range of services. Most covered elective services, prescribing and some also covered community and emergency services. Use of savings were negotiated with the PCT and could only be used to support services
2010–12	Coalition government elected, announce abolition of PCTs and establishment of CCGs	GP-led organisations with full statutory responsibility for commissioning all services other than primary care and highly specialised services. Fully established by 2012. Underspends required – annual 'efficiency' targets

for the NHS and ensure the NHS was accountable to Parliament and the public. The mandate was refreshed on an annual basis by the Secretary of State to ensure that NHSE's objectives remained up to date. An 'integrated' public health service called Public Health England (PHE), a new statutory body, was created in 2013. The aim was to provide an 'authoritative voice' on all public health issues, resulting in a better coordinated system (Department of Health, 2014). It was argued that by containing the functions of multiple organisations within one new national agency, it would reduce overlapping responsibilities and inefficiencies, and exploit synergies across services. By bringing together the knowledge and intelligence into one organisation, it was hoped that PHE would provide LAs, the DH and the NHS with clear advice and evidence on what works best in protecting and improving public health. The creation of a national body with overarching responsibility for providing public health advice and support would improve the consistency and availability of such advice.

The 2010 White Paper also advocated competition between a greater range of providers in order to produce the desired results of improved quality and greater efficiency.

The HSCA 2012 made a direct association between competitive behaviour in the NHS and competition law (Den Exter and Guy, 2014). The National Health Service Procurement, Choice and Competition Regulations No 2 2013 related to sections 75–77 and 304 (9) and (10) of the HSCA 2012, and included elements of existing guidance that were not previously subject to statutory regulation, including the PRCC and NHS procurement guidelines. These were supplemented by guidance issued by Monitor. Moreover, the Procurement, Choice and Competition Regulations indicated that competitive procurement was to be preferred. Under the HSCA 2012, Monitor had a statutory responsibility to promote competition and was obliged to carry out competition regulation with the CMA (formerly the OFT) (under the Competition Act 1998, HSCA s 72). Monitor had concurrent responsibilities with the CMA in relation to anticompetitive agreements and abuse of dominant position (HSCA s 72). Mergers involving one or more FTs were subject to the Enterprise Act 2002 (HSCA s 79) and had to be reviewed by the Competition and Markets Authority (CMA) – formerly the Office of Fair Trading (OFT) – with Monitor taking an advisory role in relation to the benefits of the merger for patients. Monitor, on the other hand, had sole responsibility for the examination of mergers between NHS Trusts. The Enterprise Act 2002 imposed a duty on the OFT to refer a merger to the Competition Commission

(CC) if it fitted the definition of a 'relevant merger situation' and if the OFT believed the merger might result in a significant lessening of competition. While Monitor was also responsible for promoting cooperation, it was the role of NHS commissioners (including CCGs), to ensure that the appropriate levels of competition and cooperation existed in their local health economies (Health and Social Care Act, 2012).

Architecture of commissioning post-HSCA 2012

Clinical Commissioning Groups (CCGs)

At the heart of the coalition government's 2010 reform was the development of *clinically led* CCGs to replace *managerially led* PCTs in commissioning healthcare for their local populations.

CCGs were required to have clinical leadership and wider clinical involvement. Hence the CCG Accountable Officer or the Chair would be a clinician. The CCG GB would also include a nurse and secondary care clinician. In addition to being clinically led (primarily GP-led), CCGs were set up as *membership organisations*. Membership was compulsory and every GP practice in England became a member of a CCG. The guidance on CCG governance (Department of Health, 2011) underlined the need to develop structures and ways of working that ensured member practices were represented and engaged. Hence CCGs were accountable to constituent GP practices (NHS England, 2012c: 3).

The HSCA 2012 handed the majority of commissioning responsibilities (such as urgent and emergency care, elective hospital care, CHS, mental health services (MHS), GP 'local enhanced services' (LES) and out-of-hours GP services) to CCGs, with the following exceptions: primary and specialist services were commissioned by NHSE; health improvement services were commissioned by LAs; and health protection and promotion services were provided by PHE (NHS Commissioning Board, 2012b).

The responsibility for commissioning primary care services (medical, dental, eye health and pharmacy) was given to NHSE to ensure a standardised model and to avoid the inherent conflict of interest that would arise from GPs commissioning themselves or their practices to provide services. From April 2015, NHSE started to devolve responsibility for commissioning primary care services to CCGs. This policy change was motivated by CCGs' knowledge of local population health needs and their assumed ability to commission integrated pathways. These benefits were seen as outweighing the risks of conflicts of interest.

CCGs were supported by CSUs, which deliver support services such as business support (for example, financial planning, human resources and information technology) and support with the commissioning cycle (for example, health needs assessment, healthcare procurement, contract negotiation and management). The provision of these services by CSUs was intended to enable CCGs to concentrate on the 'core' task of GP-led commissioning.

NHS England (NHSE)

Under the HSCA 2012, overall responsibility for running the NHS was removed from the DH and given to a new arm's length body, NHSE.

NHSE was charged with authorising CCGs, a process that entailed the submission of evidence related to a strong clinical and professional focus, patient and public engagement, good governance arrangements, collaboration and good leadership. This process was not a mere formality, with only a minority of CCGs being authorised without conditions. Following authorisation, NHSE was responsible for overseeing CCGs and assuring their performance. CCGs were subject to an annual assessment of their performance on a range of outcomes; they were also accountable to NHSE for their financial performance and spending, and they were required to comply with directions issued by NHSE and take account of documents issued by NHSE.

NHSE was given responsibility for commissioning primary care and specialised services at a national level in order to ensure standardised services and reduce variation in provision. Additionally, the commissioning of primary care services by NHSE would prevent any potential conflicts of interest for CCG members. From 2015, CCGs started to take on responsibility for commissioning primary care services with varying degrees of support from NHSE. Specialised services are those of low volume but high cost, for which risk-sharing requires planning for larger populations. NHSE commissions specialist services from 'tertiary providers'. In order to encourage the commissioning of integrated services (distinct from the new models of care outlined in the FYFV by CCGs, there has been a move towards 'collaborative commissioning' between CCGs and NHSE.

One of the key arguments made in the White Paper *Equity and Excellence* (Department of Health, 2010a) and enshrined in the legislation was of the need for greater national consistency. NHSE was set up as a single organisation with 27 Local Area Teams (LATs) organised around four 'regions'. All LATs took on direct commissioning responsibilities for GP services, dental services, pharmacy and certain aspects of optical services. There were ten LATs leading on specialised commissioning across England and a small number of LATs carrying out direct commissioning for military and prison health. In 2014, the 27 LATs (NHS Commissioning Board, 2012d) were integrated into 12 'area teams' (West and Calkin, 2014), which were further consolidated into the four 'regional teams' from April 2015.

Public Health England (PHE)

PHE was established as the national agency for public health (an executive agency to the DH) to provide leadership, coordinate health protection, deliver national campaigns, and act as a partner in local initiatives where appropriate (Department of Health, 2011b).

PHE was given four main functions: (1) to fulfil the Secretary of State's duty to protect the public's health from infectious disease and other public health hazards (for example, investigation and management of outbreaks of infectious disease, ensuring effective emergency preparedness, and resilience and response for health emergencies); (2) to secure improvements to the public's health, including reducing health inequalities; (3) to improve population health, for example, promoting the evidence on public health intervention and providing national coordination of immunisation and screening programmes; and (4) to ensure the public health system maintains the capability and capacity to tackle public health challenges.

PHE operates through four 'regions', which are coterminous with NHSE's four regional teams, and 15 'centres' (Department of Health, 2012e), which were reduced to 8 local centres plus an integrated region and centre for London (HM Government, 2017).

Local Authorities (LAs)

Local authorities were identified as key organisations to coordinate local efforts to protect and improve the public's health. The coalition government believed that strong local political leadership and better integration between health, social care and public health, would lead to a community-wide approach to protecting and promoting health and wellbeing. This was expected to realise greater opportunities and efforts to tackle the wider determinants of health at the local level, as well as tackling the individual and behavioural determinants. LAs were expected to take a broad view of what services will impact on the public's health, and to combine traditional 'public health' activities with other activity locally to maximise benefits (Department of Health (2011c).

Public Health

The public health White Paper *Healthy Lives, Healthy People* (Department of Health, 2010b) set out the government's long-term vision for the future of public health in England and aimed to create a 'wellness' service and to strengthen both national and local leadership. It emphasised that 'local government and local communities will be at the heart of improving health and wellbeing for their populations and tackling inequalities' (HM Government, 2010a). A number of fundamental changes to the structures and organisation of public health systems took effect from April 2013. The public health resources and functions of PCTs were transferred from the NHS to local government. This transfer included specialist public health staff and the budget for commissioning a range of health improvement and illness prevention services. The aim was to achieve a strengthened relationship between public health professionals and local authority (LA) personnel in all departments so that public health could be 'embedded' within all LA work to more fully address the wider determinants of health at a local level. The Director of Public Health (DPH) in a LA was expected to champion health across the whole of the LA's business.

Health and Wellbeing Board (HWB)

The HSCA 2012 gave LAs a statutory duty to create a HWB. HWBs were constituted as statutory committees of LAs with social services responsibilities and were intended to be a forum where key leaders from the health and care system worked together 'to understand their local community's needs, agree priorities and encourage commissioners to work in a more joined up way' (Department of Health, 2012a). The exact membership of HWBs was not mandated, but was subject to a minimum core membership, such as local elected representative, a representative of each CCG, DPH and a number of LA directors (adult services and children's services) (Department of Health, 2012a).

HWBs were free to expand their memberships and could choose how they wished to work.

The rationale for the creation of HWBs was to improve the health and wellbeing of the local population, reduce health inequalities and promote the integration of services. HWBs had a coordinating function across LA services, with a role in addressing the wider social determinants of health such as housing, education and planning, as well as social care.

HWBs were also expected to promote greater integration and partnership, including joint commissioning, integrated provision, and pooled budgets where appropriate. In this regard, HWBs had a statutory duty, with CCGs, to produce a Joint Strategic Needs Assessment (JSNA) and Joint Health and Wellbeing Strategy (JHWS) for their local population. They were both expected to be a 'locally owned process' to ensure that clinically led CCGs and democratically elected leaders worked together to deliver the best health and care services based on the best evidence of local needs (Department of Health, 2013b). CCGs were required to include relevant HWBs in the development and finalisation of their commissioning plans.

Table 2.2 outlines the different services commissioned by CCGs, NHSE and LAs.

Regulators

Monitor

Under the HSCA 2012, Monitor as the new economic regulator was given the most prominent role in interpreting the legal principles and advising the NHS on what behaviours were acceptable in terms of competition and cooperation (Monitor, 2014b, 2015b). Monitor (as the economic regulator for the whole of the NHS) took over some of the functions of the former CCP and, along with the national competition authorities – being, since April 2014, the CMA and prior to that the OFT and the Competition Commission – had powers to enforce competition law to prevent anticompetitive behaviour. At the same time, Monitor was also responsible for promoting cooperation (Health and Social Care Act, 2012). Monitor (2015a) maintained that delivering integrated care and complying with competition conditions were not mutually exclusive aims. It stated that it was possible to design models of care that 'give patients a choice of a provider, deliver care to individual patients in an integrated way, and enable competition

Table 2.2: List of services commissioned by CCGs, NHSE and local authorities

Services commissioned by CCGs	Services commissioned by NHSE	Public health services commissioned by LAs

• Urgent and emergency care (including 111, A&E and ambulance services)
• Out-of-hours primary medical services
• Elective hospital care
• CHS (such as rehabilitation services, speech and language therapy, and home oxygen services)
• Other community-based services (such as services provided by GP practices that go beyond the scope of the GP contract)
• Rehabilitation services
• Maternity and new-born services
• Children's healthcare services
• Services for people with learning disabilities
• MHS
• NHS continuing healthcare
• Infertility services
	• Essential and additional primary medical services through GP contract and nationally commissioned enhanced services
	• Out-of-hours primary medical services
	• Pharmaceutical services provided by community pharmacy services, dispensing doctors and appliance contractors
	• Primary ophthalmic services, NHS sight tests and optical vouchers
	• All dental services
	• Health services for people in prison and other custodial settings, members of the armed forces and their families, and prosthetics services for veterans
	• Specialised and highly specialised services
	• The following public health services:
	  — For children from pregnancy to age five (to move to LAs from 2015)
	  — Immunisation programmes
	  — National screening programmes
	  — Public healthcare for people in prison and other places of detention
	  — Sexual assault referral services
		• Tobacco control
		• Alcohol and drug misuse services
		• Obesity and community nutrition initiatives
		• Physical activity
		• Assessment and lifestyle interventions
		• Public MHS
		• Dental public health services
		• Accidental injury prevention
		• Population-level interventions to reduce and prevent birth defects
		• Behavioural and lifestyle campaigns to prevent cancer and long-term conditions
		• Local initiatives on workplace health
		• Supporting, reviewing and challenging delivery of key public health-funded and immunisation programmes
		• Sexual health services
		• Local initiatives to reduce excess deaths as a result of seasonal mortality
		• Health protection incidents and emergencies
		• Community safety, violence prevention and response
		• Local initiatives to tackle social exclusion.

*Table adapted from 'Commissioning Fact Sheet for Clinical Commissioning Groups' (NHS Commissioning Board, 2012b). Some of the services have moved or are in the process of moving: for example, primary care, specialised services.

between providers to provide services' (Monitor, 2015a). Monitor was also responsible for setting prices within the system and ensuring service continuity. In 2016 Monitor was renamed NHS Improvement (NHSI) and its remit was extended to assume regulatory powers over all types of provider to the NHS in order to facilitate market entry.

Care Quality Commission (CQC)

The Care Quality Commission (CQC) was established in 2008 as the independent regulator of health and social care providers in England. Under the HSCA 2012, the role of the CQC was strengthened as a 'quality inspectorate' across health and social care for both publicly and privately funded care (Department of Health, 2010a). Along with Monitor, the CQC was charged with issuing and overseeing the licensing of both public and private providers. In this regard, the remit of the CQC covered the essential safety and quality requirements of providers. The CQC would carry out targeted and risk-based inspections of the quality and safety of providers. Providers who failed to meet the requirements would be subject to 'enforcement action' including fines or suspension of services (Department of Health, 2010c). As with economic regulation, quality regulation of both public and private providers was intended to expedite market entry.

Contracts

Contracts were introduced into the NHS in the early 1990s as part of the internal market reforms, although they were not legally binding (Allen, 1995). Initially, there was no standard form of contract and the written documents used by commissioners varied considerably (Allen, 2002b). In 2007, a detailed form of standard contract made available by the DH for use by commissioners (Department of Health, 2009). This form of contract was designed for use with both NHS FTs and independent providers (in both of which cases it is legally binding), as well as with NHS Trusts (in which case it is not currently legally binding). The standard contract is evolving over time (Dodds, personal communication, 2011), and a new form of standard contract incorporating core commercial terms and allowing for service specifications to be agreed at local level was introduced for use in April 2013. The policy aim has been that one of the uses of contracts in the English NHS is not simply to allocate resources to providers, but as an instrument to improve services (Department of Health, 2009). One of the relevant types of contractual mechanisms is a variety of clauses aimed at achieving specified quality standards and improvements. In 2009–10 the DH introduced a quality framework called 'Commissioning for Quality and Innovation' (CQUIN), which provided financial incentives to achieve specific quality targets (Department of Health, 2008). DH guidance stated that, in addition to CQUIN, contracting parties can agree to include further financial incentives for quality improvements. There are also provisions in the standard contract which allow commissioners to impose financial penalties for breaches of nationally specified events and other aspects of poor quality care. Local commissioners can negotiate additional CQUINs and financial penalties to include in their contracts with local providers.

The HSCA 2012 made it clear that contractual relationships between commissioners (CCGs and NHSE) and a range of providers (both NHS and independent) would continue to be essential to the structure of health services in England. Quality standards developed by the National Institute for Health and Care Excellence (NICE) would inform commissioning and payment systems – thus contracts would continue to play a key role in improving quality of care. Moreover, as all NHS trusts were destined to become FTs, all contracts in respect of health services would be subject to general contract law (rather than the specific provisions originally introduced with the internal market legislation in the early 1990s).

For the first few years of the internal market, scant information was available about the costs of care, and most contracts did not contain prices of individual episodes of care. Instead, most contracts took the form of either block contracts or cost and volume contracts (Bartlett and Le Grand, 1993; Raftery et al, 1996). Block contracts amount to a fixed budget allocating the financial risks of overperformance to the provider. Cost and volume contracts involve setting the volume of cases in advance, and may lead to additional payments where the target volume of cases is exceeded, thus mitigating the risk to the provider. At the same time, contracts for limited volumes of some elective care were on a cost-per-case basis, which allocated the financial risk to the purchaser, as they could not cap their expenditure. These were made by individual GP fundholders.

Greater sophistication was introduced into pricing of acute services in 2004 by 'Payment by Results' (PbR) (Sussex and Street, 2004), and this can be regarded as an important development in the quasi-market. This prospective payment system requires care to be categorised into a series of predefined activities – called 'Healthcare Resource Groups' (HRGs), an adaptation of the Diagnosis Related Group (DRG) system developed in the United States in the 1980s. The idea of PbR was to sharpen incentives, as each episode of care reimbursed (or lost to another provider) was charged at national tariff rates, which are average costs across the whole country. This was meant to improve provider efficiency by driving down the costs of those providers whose costs are above average. PbR allocated the risk of overperformance to the purchaser, while the provider was at risk of losing income if patients were not treated in sufficient numbers (Allen, 2009a). In principle, PbR should obviate the need to negotiate prices.

Despite the fact that the NHS national standard contract set out clear rules for the allocation of financial risk through pricing of healthcare, these contractual rules may not have been followed in all cases. Although PbR appeared to be more complete in contractual terms, as prices are fixed nationally, volume of activity was not. Thus, in the context of fixed local commissioning budgets, it was possible that financial risk was managed in the local health economy in ways not foreseen by the PbR regime.

Under the HSCA, PbR was retained, and renamed the 'National Tariff', and the responsibility for setting the level of the national tariff was given to Monitor and NHSE. It has been argued that the introduction of the new regime under the HSCA would have the effect of juridifying decision making, thus removing the internal flexibility previously enjoyed by the NHS (Davies, 2013). The rationale for this was that, in order to produce a fair playing field between all types of provider (including independent ones), it was necessary for pricing rules to be transparent and applied equally to all providers. Prior to the introduction of HSCA, prices had been subject to flexibility in practice (Monitor, 2013b).

Although the HSCA 2012 envisaged that the PbR tariff would continue to be developed, many procedures were not covered by it. Some activity in acute hospitals was subject to local agreement, rather than a national price. It proved difficult to create HRGs, and thus national tariff prices, for care which is less episodic than acute hospital stays. There are still no national tariff prices for CHS or MHS (Monitor and NHS England, 2014), which are still covered by block contracts.

Developments since the HSCA

Since the HSCA 2012 took effect, there have been several important policy developments. These include (1) the FYFV (NHS England, 2014a) published in 2014; (2) Sustainability and Transformation

Plans (NHS England et al, 2015) in 2015; and (3) Accountable Care Systems (ACSs) and Accountable Care Organisations (ACOs) in 2017. All of these policies promoted the increased use of cooperative modes of coordination and downplayed the role of competition in the NHS.

Nevertheless, it should be noted that there have been no relevant legislative changes, so the HSCA 2012 provisions concerning the respective roles of NHS commissioning organisations (particularly CCGs) and the regulatory framework in respect of competition remain in force.

Five Year Forward View

The FYFV(NHS England, 2014a, 2014b), was published by NHSE in October 2014 and produced in collaboration with various stakeholders (PHE, Monitor, Health Education England, CQC, and the NHS Trust Development Authority [TDA]). The FYFV did not mention competition between organisations and instead focused on how organisations in the NHS need to cooperate with each other, and in fact at times merge to form larger organisations. It identified three 'gaps' that the NHS needed to address – the health and wellbeing gap, care and quality gap, and funding and efficiency gap. It was argued that to do this, the traditional boundaries between primary, community and secondary care would need to be dissolved. The new direction for services included: having networks of care (not just organisations); increased out-of-hospital care; greater integration of services (between primary and specialist hospital care, physical and mental health services, and health and social care); and the creation of new models of care.

The new models of care would develop more integrated care providers (ICPs) or networks of care providers to meet the needs of local people, especially those with long-term conditions and multiple health problems. 'Vanguards' were established as pilot sites for the new models of care. The first 29 Vanguards were chosen in March 2015, focusing on the following models: Multispecialty Community Providers (MCPs) – blending primary and specialist services in one organisation and multidisciplinary teams providing services in the community; Primary and Acute Care Systems (PACS) – integrating primary, hospital and MH services; and enhanced health in care homes – multi-agency support and the use of new technologies to help people stay at home. In July 2015, eight additional urgent and emergency care Vanguards were announced, focusing on developing new approaches to reduce pressure on A&E departments. A further 13 acute care collaboration Vanguards were announced in September 2015, which aimed to link hospitals to improve clinical and financial viability and reduce variations in care.

Sustainability and Transformation Plans and Partnerships

In 2015, NHSE along with other relevant NHS national bodies issued a policy document introducing the concept of local cooperative, place-based planning, known as Sustainability and Transformation Plans (NHS England et al, 2015). The guidance emphasised that this planning process would involve all 'local leaders coming together as a team, developing a shared vision with the local community, which also involves local government as appropriate; [and] programming a coherent set of activities to make it happen' (NHS England et al, 2015, page 4). Local areas were required to define their 'transformation footprint', which was needed in order to produce and deliver a local Sustainability and Transformation Plan for the period October 2016 to March 2021. In March 2016, leads for each of the Sustainability and Transformation Plan footprints were confirmed, with the majority of leaders coming from FTs/NHS Trusts (provider organisations) or CCGs (commissioning organisations) and whilst initially six leaders came from local government, by 2017 there were only two leaders from local government. These leaders, appointed by NHSE, were responsible for overseeing regional planning across the health and care system, including the reconciliation of different, often competing, interests of organisations to meet the needs of the local population. Sustainability and Transformation Plan footprints varied considerably, with each having its own strategic plan and organisational composition. Thus, for example, some Sustainability and Transformation Plan footprints included as many as 12 different CCGs while others included only one, and some have a footprint crossing LA boundaries, whilst others were coterminous with LAs.

The Sustainability and Transformation Plan process continued to be central to NHS commissioning at local level and the term Sustainability and Transformation *Plan* mutated to mean 'Sustainability and Transformation *Partnerships*' (STPs), indicating that these cooperative modes of coordination were regarded as the preferable (and in fact, mandated) method by which health services would be planned and commissioned.

Accountable and integrated care

The notion of ACO was introduced by NHSE in 2017. These were seen as natural successors to STPs under which NHS organisations would merge formally. In response to the legal obstacles to creating ACOs, including two judicial reviews, a new organisational vehicle to deliver greater integration and cooperation between providers has been proposed in the form of ACSs (NHS England, 2017c). The idea of ACSs was loosely defined and open-ended. ACSs were envisioned as an 'evolved' version of an STP, whereby NHS organisations would work together (often in partnership with LAs) as a locally integrated health system. The ACS would take on collective responsibility for resources and population health and provide more coordinated care. They would gain more control and freedom over the local health system and receive financial and regulatory support (NHS England, 2017c). In 2018, ACSs were renamed Integrated Care Systems (ICSs) (NHS England and NHS Improvement, 2018b). ICSs are expected to produce a single system operating plan and work within a single system control total (aggregate financial position). It is anticipated that over time ICSs will replace STPs (NHS England and NHS Improvement, 2018b). Chapter 9 discusses the proposed development of ICSs as outlined in the Long Term Plan (LTP) (NHS England and NHS Improvement, 2019), published in January 2019.

Looser alliance or partnership agreements between provider organisations – sometimes labelled Integrated Care Partnerships (Ham, 2018) – will be more common in ICSs as opposed to the single organisational form of an ACO. In August 2018, NHSE launched a 12-week consultation on the contracting arrangements for ICPs (formerly ACOs) (NHS England, 2018b). The purpose of the consultation was to inform NHSE's plans on whether the draft ICP contract should be further developed and if so, how it should be developed. In response to the consultation feedback, NHSE will make several changes to improve the ICP contract, before implementing it gradually, starting with a small number of commissioners (NHS England, 2019).

3

The development and early operation of Clinical Commissioning Groups (CCGs)

Anna Coleman, Imelda McDermott,
Lynsey Warwick-Giles and Kath Checkland

Introduction

The changes introduced by the HSCA 2012 represented a substantial redistribution of responsibilities within the English NHS. This included the compulsory membership of CCGs for GPs, via their practices, which was linked to a quality payment, defined locally by the CCG, for those successfully carrying out commissioning responsibilities. The policy was intentionally permissive when first introduced, with, for example, the size and composition of CCGs not imposed. In a letter to GPs in September 2010, Sir David Nicholson, Chief Executive of NHSE stated that: 'We would want to enable new organisations, and particularly [CCGs], to have the maximum possible choice of how they operate and who works for them. It is important that GP practices be given time and space to develop their plans to form commissioning consortia' (Nicholson, 2010). During October 2010, groups of GPs were invited to join aspiring CCGs, with the help of local SHAs – organisations that led the strategic development of the local health service and managed PCTs and NHS Trusts (NHS Digital, 2018) – to begin to organise themselves. By June 2011, there was over 90 per cent coverage of CCGs in England. Over time the policy became more constrained, with recommendations made for CCGs not to cross LA boundaries, optimal population coverage being suggested, and maximum management budgets being set. In supporting GP practices towards CCG establishment, NHSE published guidance setting out what should be considered when putting in place the necessary arrangements (NHS Commissioning Board, 2012c). The key elements of the guidance included:

- The need to have a defined geographical footprint in order to commission for populations not registered with a GP practice.
- The need for CCGs to be established as 'membership organisations', with GP practices as members, collectively making decisions about how the CCG should be set up and function.
- The issues to be addressed in a constitution, including: arrangements to ensure transparency; provision to hold meetings in public; appointing an audit and a remuneration committee; arrangements for relevant subcommittees if required.
- Safeguards against conflicts of interest.
- The key issues to be considered in appointing GB members, including the appointment of lay membership along with a hospital consultant and a nurse from outside the CCG's geographical area.
- The requirement for three 'leaders' within the CCG, including the need for a Chair, an Accountable Officer and a Chief Finance Officer (three at the top).
- The requirement to set up quality, audit, and remuneration committees.
- The size of the group, with large groups demonstrating how they intended to engage local practices and small groups demonstrating how they would be financially viable. Many CCGs underwent mergers – the median size after mergers (May 2012) was 235,000 population, against a median from the web survey carried out in December 2011 of 176,000, and an initial median of 163,000 in July 2011.

A timetable was set out for CCGs to apply for full authorisation as statutory bodies from July 2012, with the first CCGs taking full responsibility for commissioning the majority of care for their registered populations from April 2013.

This chapter draws upon research evidence about the establishment and early development of CCGs (2011–12). Building upon the context set out in the previous chapter, the factors affecting early CCG development are examined, highlighting the complexity of their governance structures, approaches taken to engaging with their members and the development of external relationships with a wide range of new bodies, established under the HSCA 2012. It is based on a study of developing CCGs in England conducted between September 2011 and June 2012 (Checkland et al, 2012, 2013b). The aim of the research was to explore the early experiences of emerging CCGs, investigating the factors that affected their development and to draw lessons for the future. The specific research questions addressed were:

- What have been the experiences of early CCGs over the previous 12 months?
- What factors affected their progress and development?
- What approaches were taken to:
  - being a membership organisation?
  - developing external relationships?
  - commissioning and contracting?
- What lessons could be learned for their future development and support needs?

Design and methods

This study took place in the early stages of development of CCGs and represented a snapshot of a developing situation. The data collected were both wide in scope and in-depth, going beyond sanitised accounts of CCG development to explore in greater detail the issues that arose in real time. The overall study design involved detailed qualitative case studies in eight developing CCGs, along with national web surveys at two points in time (December 2011 and April/May 2012) and telephone interviews (38, giving a 38 per cent response rate) with a random sample of CCGs. The sample of CCGs for the telephone interviews reflected the developing complexity on the ground and considered size, sociodemographic characteristics, wave of authorisation, numbers of secondary care providers, number of HWBs, closeness to previous administrative boundaries (for example, PCT, PBC Group). Qualitative data collection included: interviews with a wide variety of GPs and managers (96 in total); observation in meetings (146 meetings, 439 hours); and study of available documents. Response rates were 41 per cent and 56 per cent respectively for the web surveys. All data sources (apart from telephone interviews) were analysed together and results in this chapter represent a synthesis of the case studies and national-level data.

Case studies

Interviews

A wide range of different types of NHS manager, including those aligned to the developing CCGs and those working in PCT Clusters,

Table 3.1: Interviewees

Type of respondent	Number interviewed	Number of interviews
Managers (NHS)	47	49
GPs	33	36
Lay members	5	5
Practice managers	3	3
Nurse (clinical lead)	1	1
Others (for example, Trust manager)	1	1
LA representatives	1	1
Total	91	96

were interviewed. Interviewees included many individuals nominated for the roles of Accountable Officer and Director of Finance for the developing CCGs. Additionally clinicians (GPs, nurses), practice managers and lay representatives were interviewed (see Table 3.1).

Observations of a variety of meetings (including those at assurance level and operational level) held by the CCGs and, wherever possible, meetings between representatives of CCGs and external bodies such as service development groups; meetings with PCT clusters and shadow HWBs; and meetings between the internal governing bodies and representatives of member practices.

Documents were collected across the eight sites and included CCG governance agreements, policy statements, guidelines and accountability frameworks, as well as those associated with specific meetings (agendas, minutes, papers). These were provided in electronic format wherever possible.

More details on methods can be found in Checkland and colleagues (2012).

Results

The results focus on structure governance and autonomy; engaging CCG members; and early commissioning activity.

CCG autonomy and decision making: structures and governance

At the outset it appeared that CCGs would have significantly more autonomy than any previous clinical commissioning organisations, in that they were to be the statutory body with full budgetary responsibility. This section presents evidence relating to the development of CCGs' structures and governance procedures, in order to explore how far this autonomy and associated ability to make decisions was realised.

CCGs were instructed at the outset that they should have some sort of 'GB' with at least one nurse member, a consultant member and two lay members. The 'GB', was to be responsible for making sure 'that CCGs have appropriate arrangements in place to ensure they exercise their functions effectively, efficiently and economically and in accordance with any generally accepted principles of good governance that are relevant to it' (NHS Commissioning Board, 2012c, pages 31-32). In addition, there should be an audit committee and a remuneration committee. Over and above this it was left to individual CCGs to design their own structures, with the guidance posing a series of questions for CCGs to consider (NHS Commissioning Board, 2012c). The variation in CCG structures, in terms of their remit and functions, roles of GB members, and names used to describe committees/subgroups makes it difficult to discuss CCG structures in a general way (Checkland et al, 2016) and often made functions and responsibilities of individual parts of the governance structures opaque and difficult to understand.

Terms used within the case studies included: Board or Shadow Board; Executive or Executive Committee; Clinical Commissioning Committee; Council of Members; Forum; Collaborative; Locality; Cluster; Senate; and Cabinet. Total GB size as reported in the survey varied substantially (Checkland et al, 2012), as did membership, with some establishing a relatively small group, dominated by GPs, whilst others opened membership up to a variety of other professionals and representatives such as social service representatives and Public Health specialists. Smaller groups could at times find decision making easier to achieve, but at the expense of less engagement with the wider health and care community.

Towards the end of the study period, there was a developing consensus around the name 'GB' for the main statutory body, but still considerable variety around the naming of other subcommittees or membership groups. This made direct comparisons difficult between sites, as it was not always clear how far bodies with different names corresponded with each other. Groups were therefore identified according to their function, not their names (Table 3.2).

The distribution of functions in a given site was much more fluid than this typology suggested, with, for example, no clear separation between GB functions and more operational work, and considerable

Table 3.2: Description of groups according to function

Descriptive name	Function
'GB'	Planning to take over the statutory responsibility once authorisation was completed
Operational bodies	Including a number of different committees or workstreams and, in some sites, a formally constituted operational group, often called an 'Executive', which undertook the day-to-day management of the group's activities
Council of Members	Consisting of representatives from each practice
Locality Groups	Consisting of a smaller group of representatives from a geographical area within the CCG (not all CCGs had these)
Wider clinician groups	Two CCGs had convened a wider group of clinicians, managers and representatives from outside (for example, the LA or the local provider trust) to provide advice about a range of issues

time and effort being spent in meetings discussing which groupings should be responsible for which type of decisions. It was clear at that time that this developing complexity lay with the participants' growing awareness of the significance of the decisions they would be called on to make. As illustrated by the following quote from a manager at a larger CCG, developing governance arrangements were complex:

'Well, because we're a large CCG, if we have everybody ... so we have all of our locality chairs, and the two lay members, and the nurse representative, and the acute, um, clinician representative, all around a table, the meeting's going to be, ah, less than, um, efficient. So what I've done is created a proposal for two boards. One is the statutory board that ... What do they call it? The governing body. And the other is more of a ... It's still, to an extent, determining strategic priorities, but a subsidiary board. So you have the locality chairs on one subsidiary board comprised solely of GPs, you have a superior board – the oversight and governance board – comprised of some GP representatives from the lower board, and all those statutory appointees.' (Manager ID 60)

Further complexities arose for CCGs, in that in addition to their internal governance processes, they would also be externally accountable to the NHS Commissioning Board (renamed NHSE) and, more indirectly, to the local HWB, in ways which were still under development at the time. Together, these factors led to the development of new organisations that, although having budgetary control, could be significantly constrained in their ability to make rapid decisions or act autonomously in practice.

Engagement with members

From previous research it was known that, in a clinical commissioning organisation with decision-making power, active engagement of GPs increased the ability to achieve goals and to innovate, but this was associated with significantly increased administrative overheads (Miller et al, 2012). It was also important to consider both the meaning and practice of 'CCG ownership' and the engagement of members.

Guidance stressed the importance of GP engagement, explaining that: 'CCGs are also membership organisations, accountable to constituent GP practices' (NHS Commissioning Board, 2012a, page 3), and suggested that member practices should be actively engaged with all key decisions in setting up and operating the CCG (NHS Commissioning Board, 2012c); that is, seeing themselves as 'owners' of the CCG and of its plans. In practice, the small group of executive GPs alongside managers tended to develop constitutions, strategic plans and commissioning plans which were later submitted to the wider membership for approval. It is not always clear how far the wider GP members saw themselves as 'owning' these plans. Findings from case studies and surveys suggested that CCGs were still working out what it meant to be a membership organisation. From the case studies, some smaller CCGs were working hard to ensure that their organisations were seen as being 'owned' by their members. However, this was less obvious for the larger CCGs.

In one site, this issue was revisited in almost every meeting, and Council of Members meetings were actively used to engage the members. One GP described this process:

> 'We also have a check and balance of the Council of Members, and my feeling initially, was that meeting was far too large … there were 34 people sitting around. But in actual fact, if we watched how the conversation flowed at the last meeting, I actually felt it was really quite useful. The purpose was one, to hold us to account, but also to feed us information about what's a problem. And you saw with the Mental Health Strategy. "This is wrong." People giving both specific examples and endorsing broad feelings about how it did, and take all that in. And then go back to

the provider of that service, and say "This is what everybody is saying about it. What do you think you're going to do to change it?" So to be at that stage, is actually really quite exciting because it's almost showing how we're going to operate in the future.' (GP ID 283)

It is clear from this quote that this GP saw the GB as being 'held to account' by the membership. However, in the following quote, a manager from a different site argues that the Council of Members had given the Executive the power to make decisions, upon which the wider membership could then comment, rather than the wider membership owning the decisions. In other words, the Executive would be required to give an account to their membership, without necessarily being accountable in a more direct sense:

'Yes, that … I suppose that really is they have given the exec team responsibility [to] decide, you know, that direction and the plan, so your first signoff is with the exec team, but then you take it to the wider group to say this is what we're going to take forward to see what we can develop, you know, what do you want to do, so it's just really exposing it to the wider remit as a sort of communication exercise really, but also it's their then chance to say you're all barking up the wrong tree; this is not right, that sort of thing.' (Manager ID 42)

All case study CCGs were in the process of deciding how they should engage with their members in the longer term. Many different modes of communication and engagement were planned, such as newsletters or briefings sent round to all GPs and intranet sites. Communication with the membership (that is, GP practices) was seen as important by all case study CCGs. Three different approaches to communication were identified:

- as predominantly a one-way process, focused upon 'informing' the membership;
- as a limited two-way process, with the emphasis upon both informing the membership and capturing 'usable intelligence' from the clinical front line;
- as a full two-way process, focused upon capturing the views of the membership to set the direction of the group as well as on keeping them informed.

Although CCGs had no formal role to performance manage membership practices, case study sites experienced a tension between wanting to engage with their membership practices and being in a position to potentially challenge practices about actions and decisions being made that could impact on commissioning decisions. A significant challenge was trying to ensure that member practices adhered to CCG policies without any formal contractual mechanisms to hold the practices to account (these were held by NHSE). Although official documents referred to a more supportive CCG role to improve the quality of local primary care services, examples from case study sites demonstrated that CCGs were carrying out more performance management roles, which included practices being compared against each other with regard to particular indicators and practices such as poorly performing practices working with comparable well-performing practices, to improve primary care services.

The role, purpose and remit of Locality groups remained unclear, especially for those groups which had undergone a merger. There was a lack of clarity over the extent to which Locality groups should have responsibility for budgets and for commissioning decisions. The performance management of practice behaviour relating to commissioning such as referrals and prescribing was viewed as a legitimate role for CCGs, often building on work already started in sites. However, a potential tension between the desire to be a meaningful membership organisation and the perceived need to manage performance was evident.

These findings suggested that what it means to 'engage' grassroots GPs in CCGs was yet to be clearly formulated. The meaning of 'membership', the extent to which grassroots GPs are expected to 'own' the agenda, the purpose of 'communication' and the role of Locality groups all still needed careful consideration and 'engagement' may mean different things in groups of different sizes.

Commissioning activity

At the time of the research, CCGs had not taken formal responsibility for commissioning and contracting. Unlike all previous manifestations of GP-led commissioning, CCGs would ultimately be given full responsibility for virtually the entire commissioning budget with the exception of primary care. Respondents in the case study sites were very much aware of the implications of this, and of the challenges ahead:

'There is no longer going to be a PCT to pick up the pieces. We are going to have to hold each other to account (localities and GPs) and work hard at this. Localities need to own contracts. We have to look at financial credibility. We have an overall limit and only have the small transitional fund to fall back on. We need to be on top of things from quarter one and decide how we are going to monitor things.' (Extract from field notes executive meeting March 2012 M30)

In this context it was found that most case study sites had been through some sort of prioritisation process for commissioning, which informed their ongoing strategic plan. In the second survey, three-quarters of CCGs had already set up new services, or planned to do so in the next 12 months, and two-fifths had changed or planned to change some providers of existing services. Most changes to services reported by the survey respondents and observed in the case study sites had been small-scale, short-term pilots or linked to LES or innovation funding and only small-scale decommissioning had occurred, if at all. Some GB members in the case study CCGs appeared to recognise the need to take as broad a view as possible of the commissioning task, moving away from small-scale, practice-level interventions:

'for me it's really amazing to watch these clinicians leading change on a really significant scale, and it's very different to, I guess, what I thought might happen, after seeing those early stages of practice-based commissioning, which were, you know, doing a little bit of dermatology in your practice, for other practices, it was very small scale.' (Manager ID 204)

Commissioning was in transition and tensions could be seen between the various levels of organisation (PCT Clusters, CCGs and Localities) in some areas. Many of the case study sites made claims about the 'added value' of having clinicians (almost exclusively GPs) involved in both commissioning and contracting. This will be further discussed in Chapter 4. There were some issues caused by time constraints faced by GP commissioners (for example, CCG work versus seeing patients), and case study GPs were beginning to realise that their new role would mean taking on greater responsibility and accountability for commissioning decisions for their local populations.

Engaging more widely (with public health, HWBs and other LA services such as education, housing and so on) was seen to be a key aspect of development for CCGs if they were to make changes broader than those at practice level for their populations. A further key area in which the case study CCGs felt that CCGs would add value and 'do things differently' from previous GP-led commissioning schemes was in the area of negotiating with providers:

> 'We're beginning to see some successes in terms of GPs' involvement in some of the, some of the contracting rounds, so ... They actually go along to the Contracting meetings. And, you know, and giving clinical view and clinical input around some of those discussions and conversations. And that can add real value in terms, for both the providers and the commissioners, to really start driving forwards some of those tricky conversations.' (Manager ID 5)

With the whole system in flux, a lot of hard work was being undertaken by GPs and managers involved in the establishment and early operation of CCGs, and ongoing changes affected the emerging CCGs themselves, as well as the wider context around them. Generally there was support for the idea of GP-led commissioning and some claims about the added value that GPs could bring to the contracting process (knowledge of patients and their needs locally – discussed further in Chapter 4). It was generally agreed that other clinicians had little involvement overall because of the many changes happening all at once due to the HSCA 2012, disruption and confusion could be seen at all levels of the system. GP involvement in commissioning had already been strengthened prior to these changes, however, and a number of respondents expressed the belief that many of the objectives of the HSCA 2012 changes could have been achieved within existing structures, that is, PCTs alongside PBC groups (this will be further discussed in Chapter 4).

Conclusion

This chapter has discussed some of the challenges faced by CCGs in their early period of establishment. There were a number of tensions highlighted within the developing policy context of the time. This included the need for clarity over which aspects of such a programme were open to modification and which were constrained by higher level strategic decisions and legislation as well as clarity and timeliness of published guidance to support developments – whilst organisations did not want to be directed from above, they appreciated early clarity of what the eventual overall structure should look like, with clear guidance as to what was and was not 'allowed'. Within this clear structure organisations liked to be given the autonomy to innovate and develop their own local organisational responses, given specific local circumstances. Organisations also wanted greater clarity of the relationships and accountabilities between different bodies, such as CCGs and NHSE while personal contacts between organisations across health and care were valued, especially at times of flux.

It was found that the history of previous commissioning structures and arrangements played an important role in the development of each CCG, as did the approach taken by local leaders and by the Primary Care Trust or Cluster and the developing NHSE local team (Miller et al, 2012). Engagement with local bodies such as HWBs and LAs were also significantly affected by local history, prior relationships and geography. The approach taken by NHSE to CCG development, with early freedom to develop as they chose increasingly curtailed by more prescriptive guidance and a complex assurance regime, led to some frustrations for those involved.

It has previously been shown that clinical involvement in commissioning is most effective when GPs felt able to act autonomously. Complicated internal structures, developed alongside external accountability relationships, meant that CCGs freedom to act became more constrained over time. Effective GP engagement was important in determining outcomes of clinical commissioning, and at the time this research was undertaken, there were a number of issues that CCGs still had to consider, including: who felt they had 'ownership' of the CCG; how internal communication was conceptualised and being played out; and the role and remit of Locality groups. Previous forms of GP-led commissioning had tended to focus on local services and services provided in primary care. However, CCGs had ambitions beyond this. Using approaches developed under PBC, CCGs had ambitions to improve the quality in their constituent practices. Significant factors at the time of CCG development included constrained managerial support and the ability to encourage and maintain effective GP engagement.

In relation to being a membership organisation, engagement of GPs and ownership, CCGs needed to pay attention to their membership, including the roles which Locality groups and the wider Council of Members play. As CCGs were developing, their ability to change GP behaviour depended upon their perceived legitimacy, which in turn depended upon the approach that they took to engaging members. The research suggested that CCGs needed to consider: the degree of autonomy devolved to Localities; the role of the members in contributing to strategy development; approaches to quality improvement/performance management; and the extent to which the CCG may be a vehicle for the transfer of expertise and resources between practices. In addition, to help ensure the development of a new generation of clinical leaders, resources could usefully be devoted to encouraging a model of incremental engagement that builds upon GPs' commitment to local clinical innovation.

With regard to commissioning activity and wider relationships in the developing system, CCGs had ambitions to make changes to the wider system, not just their own GP practices and services. However, there was ongoing uncertainty of how best to link up effectively with fledgling HWBs and public health, both now located in LAs. In some sites there was a clear desire to 'embed' public health at GB level, whereas others saw it more in terms of public health offering a service to the CCG. The one area in which the case study sites felt that GPs could really make an impact was in engagement with providers around service development and contracting; although at the time of the research it remained to be seen whether this involvement yielded positive impacts in the longer term that go beyond the needs and concerns of practices. Many areas were yet to be fully explored, with the research taking place at the very early stages of development. Data represented a snapshot in time and as a result further PRUComm research followed up some of these areas of interest. These included questions around:

- How can the need for autonomy and efficient decision making be reconciled with the need for robust internal governance processes?
- How tightly would the NHS Commissioning Board (renamed NHSE from 1 April 2013) seek to monitor and performance manage CCGs, and what would be the impact of this?
- What would it mean for practices in the longer term to be a 'member' of a CCG?
- Would CCGs have the legitimacy required to intervene in their members' practices to improve quality?
- Would CCGs continue to be seen as legitimate by their members, once they assume responsibility for making difficult decisions?
- What would be the role and function of locality groups in the longer term?
- How would CCGs work with the new public health system, and would they make the transition to focusing on wider issues of population health?

- Would concerns about conflicts of interest hamper the development of new services in practices (traditionally a strength of GP-led commissioning)? (Checkland et al, 2013b)

The following chapters will take forward the further development of CCGs, looking at clinical involvement in greater depth (Chapter 4) and the additional responsibilities associated with primary care co-commissioning (Chapter 5).

4

Clinical engagement in commissioning: past and present

*Kath Checkland, Anna Coleman, Imelda McDermott,
Rosalind Miller, Stephen Peckham, Julia Segar,
Stephen Harrison and Neil Perkins*

Introduction

As discussed in Chapters 1 and 2, one of the central tenets of the HSCA 2012 was the desirability of increasing the involvement of GPs (and other clinicians) in the commissioning of services for their patients. This ideological commitment – based upon belief and founded, in part at least, upon an implicit denigration of managerial work (in order to increase control over the NHS and commissioners), had far-reaching consequences in the design of the reforms. For example, the initial separation of responsibility for commissioning primary care services from secondary and community services was deemed necessary because of the potential for conflicts of interest, whilst the creation of CCGs as 'membership organisations' had, as seen in Chapter 3, significant implications for their organisation and governance. The initial White Paper, 'Equity and Excellence' (Department of Health, 2010a: 9) was relatively non-specific about the expected benefits of clinical leadership of commissioning. It was argued that:

> The headquarters of the NHS will not be in the Department of Health or the new NHS Commissioning Board but instead, power will be given to the front-line clinicians and patients. The headquarters will be in the consulting room and clinic. The Government will liberate the NHS from excessive bureaucratic and political control, and make it easier for professionals to do the right things for and with patients, to innovate and improve outcomes.

The document suggested that the proposals would: 'liberate professionals and providers from top down control'; shift decision making closer to patients; enable better dialogue between primary and secondary care practitioners; and ensure that service development had real clinical involvement. However, the mechanisms underlying these perceived benefits were unstated. Furthermore, it was claimed that, whilst previous incarnations of GP-led commissioning (which in the UK go back to the creation of 'GP fundholding' in the 1990s) had delivered some benefits, these had been limited by the failure to give those involved complete autonomy and real budgets. The creation of CCGs, it was argued, would remedy these problems and 'liberate' clinicians to significantly improve care.

This chapter examines these claims in more detail. The first section explores the history of clinical involvement in commissioning in the UK, setting out the previous structures and processes by which clinical involvement was procured and managed. It looks at the evidence relating to these previous schemes, via a systematic review of the relevant literature, and then describes the detailed study of the involvement of clinicians in CCGs, using a realist approach to explore the contexts and mechanisms underlying observed outcomes. Finally, the chapter discussion returns to the claims made about clinical involvement in commissioning and consider them against the evidence have presented. In particular, it is considered how far the establishment of CCGs as statutory budget-holding bodies was necessary in order to secure clinical involvement, and whether the further development of previous structures could have delivered equivalent – or greater – benefits.

The history of GP-led commissioning in the NHS

Since the introduction of the purchaser–provider split there have been initiatives in the NHS to try to increase the engagement of GPs in the process of planning and purchasing services (see Table 2.1). In part this reflects the design of the UK health system: GPs are the 'gatekeepers' to more specialised services, with access to specialised care only available upon referral. In such a system, hospital activity represents the sum total of the referral decisions made by individual GPs; controlling both the cost and volume of specialised activity requires GPs to consider carefully the need for referral, and to be aware of the costs of their decisions.

Beyond the UK NHS, other health systems have experimented with some forms of GP involvement in purchasing services. The most well-established primary care organisations outside of England can be found in New Zealand in the form of independent practitioner associations and community health organisations (Smith and Mays, 2007). On a smaller scale, in Europe, Estonia, Catalonia and the former Soviet Union have introduced schemes allowing clinicians to hold budgets. For example, in Catalonia, doctors and nurses hold budgets for defined populations of around 50,000–100,000 in order to cover primary health centre costs, diagnostic tests and specialist referrals (Figueras et al, 2005b). Approaches to primary care purchasing range from the exercise of professional influence – advising the main purchaser – to active purchasing where GPs have autonomy with budgetary control (McCallum et al, 2006). It is beyond the scope of this chapter to explore these alternative approaches. However, the existence of such schemes across different health systems suggests that the issues which drive interest in the engagement of frontline clinicians with the details of purchasing decisions are universal.

Evidence from the past

In order to understand in more depth the issues surrounding clinical engagement in commissioning, a systematic review of the evidence from the evaluation of these schemes in the UK was undertaken. This section is based upon an account of the findings of the literature review, published in 2015 (Miller et al, 2015). The research addressed the question: what happens when GPs engage in commissioning? It specifically explored:

1. The roles played by clinicians in commissioning.
2. The nature of clinical engagement in the commissioning process.
3. The extent to which clinicians could exercise control and influence over commissioning decisions.
4. The impact of clinical engagement on:
   - the ability to effect patterns of care;
   - changing primary care practice including prescribing and performance management;
   - quality and patient experience;
   - financial issues such as costs versus savings and the awareness of costs;
   - relationships within commissioning groups and with other agencies.

The research built upon a systematic review carried out between October 2009 and August 2010 (Newman et al, 2012). Of the 600 studies identified, 339 were concerned with health. In March 2011 an electronic literature search was conducted in 'social policy and practice', 'Econlit', 'Medline', 'PsychINFO' and 'CINAHL' following the same search strategy used in the previous review. In addition, three key journals, and the bibliographies of key reviews on primary care commissioning (Mays et al, 2001; Smith et al, 2004; Mannion, 2008) were hand-searched, and any relevant papers from formal evaluations of previous GP-led commissioning schemes (Mays et al, 1998a; Bevan et al, 1999; Smith et al, 2000; Coleman et al, 2009; Regen et al, 2001) were also examined. This search yielded an additional 175 references. The methods used in the review are described fully in the project report (Miller et al, 2012). In total 218 papers were included, and assessed using a standard data extraction tool. These were then used to construct a number of evidence matrices and identified themes, based upon the research questions.

Evidence about the nature of clinical involvement in the commissioning process

Firstly, the nature of clinical involvement in the commissioning process was explored, including: the type of roles assumed by clinicians; attitudes of clinicians towards the different schemes and their motivations for joining; the dynamic between clinical leaders and the wider clinical body; the level of clinical control over commissioning decisions; and the perceived level of influence over external organisations.

In all of the schemes that were examined, GPs (rather than other practice employees) tended to take the lead, sometimes working with designated business managers (British Medical Association, 1997; Hine and Bachmann, 1997; Surender and Fitzpatrick, 1999). Each new clinical commissioning scheme generated differing levels of engagement, and this engagement was driven by differing motivations depending upon the focus of the scheme. For example, fundholding enabled 'entrepreneurial' GPs to generate investment in their practices (with this effect most marked in so-called 'early adopters'), whilst engagement in alternative schemes tended to be driven by hostility to fundholding (Ennew et al, 1998; Wyke et al, 2001). However, involvement in all schemes tended to be driven by a sense from those involved that GPs were better informed about patient needs than managers, as they had practice-level data and direct feedback from patients on healthcare services (Dixon et al, 1998; Wyke et al, 2001; Coleman et al, 2009).

In all commissioning models, the ability to innovate was cited as a key motivator (Mays et al, 2001; Smith et al, 2004; Mannion, 2008), and this was determined by the extent to which those involved enjoyed autonomy over such things as decisions about services, and the allocation of budgets. The evaluation of TPP found that those groups given the most autonomy were those most likely to be innovative in terms of changes made (Mays et al, 1998b). However, where autonomy was restricted this limited the degree of influence or the extent of influence and this was likely to create less engagement by the wider body of GPs and clinicians (Mays et al, 1998a; Cowton and Drake, 1999a, 1999b). Involvement in commissioning could generate increased engagement, with those taking leading roles reporting increased commitment over time (Mays et al, 1998a; Coleman et al, 2009). However, such engagement requires clinicians to invest significant amounts of time which would otherwise have been spent seeing patients (Howie et al, 1993).

Clinical engagement in commissioning reached a historical low point with the introduction of PCTs in 2003, with few GPs involved in any way (Bate et al, 2007). GPs cited heavy workloads and time constraints as barriers to more involvement, and reported that they were marginalised in key decision-making processes (Regen et al, 2001). With the introduction of PBC, clinical engagement improved but devolved decision making was often nominal – especially regarding budgetary decisions (Checkland et al, 2011). The national evaluation of TPPs found that GPs were willing to participate in the management of a budget (Place et al, 1998). Thus, real responsibility and control over the budget does appear to be possible and accepted by GPs, although generally the evidence suggests that in all manifestations of GP-led commissioning only a small handful of GPs ever get involved in this aspect of commissioning (Malbon and Mays, 1998).

In summary, evidence from past GP-led commissioning schemes suggested that a key determinant of clinical engagement was the extent to which GPs felt that they had some autonomy and control to respond to what they perceived were key issues that affected their patients' experience of healthcare. Where autonomy was granted and 'success' experienced, engagement grew, but where there was less perceived autonomy and control, GPs tended to disengage (Wilkin et al, 2001; Bate et al, 2007). In past schemes the attitude of the 'parent' commissioning body was a key factor, with those prepared to cede control and support clinical commissioners to act being rewarded with increased commitment by GPs. While not all GPs were active supporters of those GPs who engaged with, or participated in, commissioning, maintaining wider clinical engagement was felt to be a priority by those leading schemes but the extent to which this was achieved varied considerably (Bravo Vergel and Ferguson, 2006; Coleman et al, 2009). Engagement was easier in smaller schemes but these tended to be limited in scope while more comprehensive schemes found it more difficult to engage with a wider GP community.

Engagement and outcomes

The evidence as to the impact of GP-led commissioning was examined. This was variable in scope and quality. There was most evidence related to those areas which were easiest to measure, such as changes in prescribing (Bradlow and Coulter, 1993; Surender and Fitzpatrick, 1999; Wilson et al, 1999; Walker and Mathers, 2002), waiting times (Kammerling and Kinnear, 1996; Dowling, 1997; Propper et al, 2002), referrals (Mays et al, 1998a; Croxson et al, 2001; Dusheiko et al, 2006; Coleman et al, 2009) and specific service changes (Corney and Kerrison, 1997; Redfern and Bowling, 2000; Drummond et al, 2001). Success in making change happen in these areas appeared to be related, in part, to peer review of performance. Thus, where rank-and-file GPs were engaging with the commissioning organisation, their behaviour could be more easily influenced, and this was generally easier in smaller organisations (Glennerster et al, 1994a; Coleman et al, 2009).

Overall, the areas with the most convincing evidence of success in making changes happen included reductions in prescribing costs and reduced waiting times (Coleman et al, 2009; Mays et al, 1998a; Smith et al, 2000). However, some studies raised questions about issues of equity (Glennerster et al, 1994a; Kammerling and Kinnear, 1996).

Others claimed positive outcomes relating to the development of services at the community level, both within practices, such as in-house physiotherapy clinics, and at the interface between primary and secondary care, such as creation of a discharge liaison officer (Glennerster et al, 1994a; Hine and Bachmann, 1997; Goodwin et al, 1998; Regen et al, 2001; Wyke et al, 2001). Unfortunately, there was little critical appraisal or evaluation of these new services and the benefits they conferred was therefore unclear. In many cases, these developments were not accompanied by the necessary resource shifts out of secondary care, indicating that there was service duplication and the cost-effectiveness remained doubtful. Areas chosen for development were mostly not informed by needs assessment or user engagement but were chosen on the basis of GP interest or perceived local need (Mays, 1996).

Little evidence was found of success in changing secondary care services, although where this was the main focus of GP-led commissioning groups, some changes to the pattern of acute hospital use were achieved (Drummond et al, 2001; Craig et al, 2002). Few GPs were interested in wider, large-scale, population-based commissioning (Mays et al, 1998a; Coleman et al, 2009; Checkland et al, 2011). While improving the quality of care for their patients was a prime motivator for many GPs to engage in commissioning (Glennerster et al, 1994b), there was little convincing empirical evidence to suggest that any of the GP-led commissioning schemes improved the overall quality of care for patients (Lapsley et al, 1997; Redfern and Bowling, 2000). Neither was there evidence that GP commissioners prioritised or addressed issues of quality of secondary care services, although research into PBC suggested that the development of commissioning networks had provided a mechanism for supporting quality development in general practice (Coleman et al, 2009). In terms of the factors enabling success, more GP engagement seemed to lead to more success in achieving goals and stated objectives. This was a common finding across GP fundholding, TPP and PBC (Mays et al, 1998a; Surender and Fitzpatrick, 1999; Coleman et al, 2009; Checkland et al, 2011). However, in larger schemes such as TPP this engagement was expensive. Place and colleagues' (1998) study of seven TPPs found that more than 50 per cent of the incremental cost associated with TPPs (compared to purchasing as fundholders) was committed to managing internal relations – that is, coordinating the views of independent GPs and involving them in the commissioning process (Place et al, 1998). The benefits of increased engagement must therefore be weighed against these higher transaction costs. Across the schemes there was also evidence that sufficient management resources were paramount and, further, that higher management costs were associated with greater success (Posnett et al, 1998).

Summary

In summary, review of the evidence found that it is possible to engage GPs in the commissioning of services, and that there was some evidence that such schemes may have an impact on such things as prescribing costs and waiting times. However, no clear evidence was found to suggest that involving GPs in commissioning led to improvements in population health. It was observed that there were 'virtuous cycles', where successful engagement of GPs which led to local action generated greater local engagement, and 'vicious cycles', where clinicians withdrew from engagement if they felt they had no influence. The environment within which GP-led commissioners operated was very important in determining whether they were successful. Where there was a more permissive and supportive environment, GP-led commissioners were generally more able to achieve both their stated objectives. Internal relationships between the clinical leaders and membership were also key to successful initiatives. Continued support from the wider clinician body was important in terms of sustaining the legitimacy of commissioning actions by the leading clinicians and in ensuring that the membership bought in to any changes that they were required to make at their practice. Finally, it was clear from the review that GP-led commissioning had tended to focus on activities that were seen as most relevant to primary care, including addressing prescribing and developing primary and community care services. There was little evidence that GP clinicians had changed secondary care services or that clinical involvement in commissioning had led to any particular outcome.

GP 'added value' in CCGs

As discussed in the introduction, the engagement of GPs and other clinicians in the commissioning of services is not based upon any particular body of evidence or theory. Rather, it is an ideological approach which reading of the relevant policy documents suggests arises out of an implicit belief in the limitations of management and managers (Learmonth, 1997). During the early phases of the research on CCGs (see Chapter 3) it was repeatedly claimed that putting GPs in leadership positions for commissioning was important, but the rationale underlying this was often vague and non-specific. A more in-depth study was therefore undertaken, exploring the 'added value' that GPs brought to the commissioning process. This section of the chapter is based upon a paper published in the *Journal of Health Services Research and Policy* in 2016 (McDermott et al, 2016a).

Design and methods

Using realist evaluation (Pawson, 2013) (see Chapter 1) as a framework, seven of the case study sites used in the earlier research on CCG development (see Chapter 3) were revisited. An initial phase of investigation involved 42 interviews with clinicians and managers (Table 4.1).

The focus of these interviews was on the programme theories (see Chapter 1) held by respondents as to how clinical involvement in commissioning would 'add value' to the process. These programme

Table 4.1: Interview respondents by site and type

Site	Type of respondent		
	GPs	Managers	Nurse (clinical lead)
Site 1	7	0	0
Site 2	7	0	0
Site 4	4	0	0
Site 5	5	1	0
Site 6	3	1	1
Site 7	2	0	0
Site 8	7	4	0
Total: 42	35	6	1

theories were then refined and developed in observation of CCG meetings in four case study sites. As is often the case, initial programme theories were broad and lacking in detail. In particular, the accounts provided limited consideration of the contextual conditions which might support or inhibit the realisation of any advantages associated with GP-led commissioning. In order to investigate this further a range of different types of CCG meetings, such as the GB, executive groups, membership and informal group meetings, were attended in each site. Observation was made of who was in the room, the extent to which clinical knowledge was mobilised, and clinician–manager interactions. A total of 48 meetings were attended (approximately 111 hours of observations). The realist approach adopted requires the further elaboration of the initial programme theories identified, ascertaining the contexts and the mechanisms under which theories did or did not appear to lead to beneficial outcomes (Pawson, 2013). In this case the 'outcomes' sought were evidence of clinical knowledge being mobilised in some way.

Programme theories: how do GPs 'add value' to commissioning?

In the initial interviews, four 'programme theories' were identified underlying the claims about GP 'added value' in commissioning:

- Theory 1: GPs' frontline knowledge about patient experiences would enable them to identify problems and deal with them promptly.

- Theory 2: GPs' frontline knowledge about services would enable them to improve service design.
- Theory 3: GPs' clinical experience and knowledge would enable them to have the authority to speak to other clinicians in ways which improve commissioning.
- Theory 4: GPs and managers have a symbiotic relationship, which together is more than the sum of its parts, and hence enhances the commissioning process.

Clinical leadership and decision making

Theory 1 (GPs' knowledge about patient experiences) and Theory 2 (GPs' knowledge about services)

The interviewees suggested that GPs' frontline knowledge about patients and available services would enable them to identify and deal with problems early and improve service design. These theories were consonant with claims made about all of the previous incarnations of GP-led commissioning. In practice it was found that it was not a foregone conclusion that such knowledge would be brought forward and used in the commissioning process. In particular, it was found that, whilst specific local knowledge about patient needs and services could be useful, commissioning decisions also required access to aggregated formal data, and that the format and conduct of CCG meetings could significantly affect the extent to which GPs were able to engage and mobilise their knowledge. Important issues included:

- A facilitative meeting environment, with good chairing and positive encouragement to contribute.
- Proactive communication with clinicians in advance of meetings in order to ensure that clinicians were aware of the issues to be decided. Their effectiveness was enhanced if they were given specific tasks within the meetings, such as a particular area of a topic to lead on, or a question to ask.
- A willingness to be flexible and to vary meeting formats.

In the latter case, one meeting was observed in which a 'select committee enquiry' format was adopted. Clinicians were prepared in advance with specific areas in which to ask questions, and provider representatives appeared as 'expert witnesses' to explain aspects of their services and of the particular commissioning issues being discussed. By contrast, in another site a meeting was observed between commissioners and providers convened to discuss problems associated with the ambulance service. Whilst prior to the meeting clinicians had voiced a number of significant concerns, in the meeting itself clinicians appeared too diffident to raise their concerns.

CCGs were established as membership organisations, with individual GP practices designated as members. However, this fact alone was not enough to facilitate active GP engagement. It was found that CCGs needed to actively seek out the views and experiences of the wider GP and clinician community. This was difficult, with all of the case study sites struggling to find effective ways of engaging their member practices.

The interviewees also claimed that GPs' position on the frontline allowed them to 'see the whole system'. However, the observations showed that GPs' knowledge was often very specific – that is, pertinent to a particular service – and they did not necessarily have insights into a full range of services, or about how services worked in general. Service reconfiguration and a proliferation of providers made it very difficult for individuals to understand the full range of services available locally. The sites recognised this, with many seeking to establish some kind of searchable database which pulled together information on the range of available services. Overall, clinical voices were valuable in providing contextual details and information as to whether services were actually being delivered as intended, but they required additional information from managers in order to understand fully the pattern of available services.

Policy rhetoric presented CCGs as different from previous initiatives because GPs in CCGs would take full commissioning responsibility, with CCGs as the responsible statutory bodies (Department of Health, 2010a). In practice, it was found that, in some ways, GP involvement in CCGs looked very similar to GP involvement in previous GP-led commissioning. In particular, most GP leaders who were actively engaged in CCGs held some sort of leadership role in the past, with many involved with fundholding, TPP and PBC. However, while previously clinical involvement was generally limited to those in leadership positions, in CCGs, by contrast, clinical involvement occurred at different levels of the organisation. Some CCGs had 'Localities', 'Neighbourhoods' or a formal 'Council of Members' who were or were not given devolved budgets and responsibility. Thus, unlike previous initiatives, clinical input and decision making occurred at various different levels in different CCGs. This made it difficult to draw general conclusions about GP involvement as the extent to which the new system had enabled better or more robust GP involvement varied in different CCGs.

Theory 3 (clinician-to-clinician discussions)

Participants from the case study sites said they felt that CCGs had enabled GPs to become more involved in contracting, and that having GPs involved in contracting meetings with providers enabled clinician-to-clinician discussions, and having clinicians leading the process made provider clinicians more likely to engage. This theory suggested that GPs contributed significantly to commissioning because their clinical experience gave them knowledge and experience which they could use to speak to other clinicians in ways which improved commissioning. GPs' clinical experience gave them the authority to talk about clinical issues, and to challenge providers if required, in a way that managers could not.

In seeking to explore this theory, it seemed likely that most of this type of GP involvement would occur in pathway development and contracting meetings. However, in spite of attendance at many such meetings, not many instances were observed in which commissioning clinicians brought their clinical knowledge to bear in challenging their provider colleagues; indeed, some of the case study CCGs made a conscious decision for managers to lead such meetings, as it was felt that they did not represent a good use of GPs' time. This suggested that the claims made by those espousing this theory – that clinicians brought a unique and important focus to meetings with providers – was not much experienced in practice. A few instances were observed in which GPs were actively involved in challenging providers and holding them to account, but this only occurred when there was careful preparation of the GPs, with clear roles assigned to those present.

Theory 4 (clinician–manager symbiosis)

Participants also claimed that GPs and managers had a symbiotic relationship which together was more than the sum of its parts. By 'symbiosis' is meant that the relationship enabled both parties to work much more effectively than they would have been able to do alone. Managers would formulate and write strategies, business plans, and provide a systematic overview of the range of services while GPs would assist in clinical input and engage with other clinicians. Mechanisms which enable this theory to work include a history of working together. However, it was also found that where this history did not exist, careful appointment procedures in which GPs were fully engaged could support the development of new close working relationships. It was also important that both GPs and managers recognised that they had different skills and contributions and that they felt able to challenge one another. The status of the CCG as a membership organisation was crucial and so is the confidence that GP membership have towards the GP–manager team working on their behalf. The experience of 'success' and having a joint responsibility for programme delivery was important both in developing the close and supportive relationship between the two individuals and in bringing the wider membership along with the process.

Summary

In summary, it was hard to identify clear evidence in the case studies of specific 'added value' provided by the presence of GPs in leadership roles in CCGs. Whilst there were some specific instances where GPs' knowledge or experience was valuable in the pursuit of a particular outcome, this did not occur routinely, rather it required specific conditions. In particular, it was found that adequate preparation of GP leaders prior to meetings, with clear roles assigned, and active approaches to the engagement of GPs beyond the GB were important. It was also found that close relationships between GPs and managers were established in many CCGs, and these could be facilitative in achieving the organisation's aims. Experience of 'success' was important in reinforcing commitment.

Conclusion

Enabling clinical leadership – specifically leadership by GPs – was one of the key underlying aims of the HSCA 2012. There have been numerous attempts to do this in the past, and the literature review showed that, whilst it was possible to engage GPs in commissioning, there was little evidence that this led to large-scale change in health service delivery. GP involvement tended to be most successful when focused upon small-scale changes, particularly those aspects of services most pertinent to general practice. There was some evidence that GP involvement can have an impact on the quality of primary care service delivery, but less evidence of any impact on population health or on larger-scale service delivery. The realist approach allowed for in-detail exploration of the extent to which espoused 'programme theories' on clinical involvement in commissioning would generate improved outcomes. It was found that, whilst it was possible for GPs to influence the commissioning process, this did not occur automatically, requiring specific preparation and careful management. This is in keeping with the findings of other research in this area. For example, Story and colleagues explore GP leadership in CCGs, finding that, whilst some successful 'GP leadership' was observed, this occurred in limited circumstances (Storey et al, 2018). Towards the end of this phase of the research (in 2014) it was announced that CCGs would take over delegated responsibility for the commissioning of primary care services. This development would seem to be consonant with the evidence from the review of the literature related to clinical involvement in commissioning, namely the fact that clinical involvement appeared to be most effective in relation to services provided in a community setting, and that peer-review of the quality of primary care services delivered could support service improvement. The next chapter explores in more depth the process by which CCGs took on these extra responsibilities.

5

Commissioning primary care services: concepts and practice

*Imelda McDermott, Kath Checkland, Anna Coleman,
Lynsey Warwick-Giles, Stephen Peckham, Donna Bramwell,
Valerie Moran and Oz Gore*

Introduction

Under the HSCA 2012, NHSE was responsible for commissioning primary care services. However, in 2014 CCGs were invited to volunteer to take on responsibility for commissioning services from their member GP practices in addition to their wider responsibilities for commissioning acute and community services. This chapter draws upon research into the establishment of the 'co-commissioning' of primary care services by CCGs, which was conducted from April 2015 to April 2017 (McDermott et al, 2018). This chapter starts by exploring the history of primary care commissioning and financing in England and discusses the broad policy objectives which underpinned this significant change in CCGs' role and scope. It examines whether and how the policy intention works in practice and explores factors affecting development of the policy, highlighting concerns over conflicts of interest, challenges in implementing the policy and unintended consequences. For clarity, the term 'primary care commissioning' is employed because this is the term used throughout the relevant policy documents. While globally the term 'primary care' often refers to the full range of out-of-hospital services, including community nursing and so on, in the UK, for the purposes of commissioning, a distinction is usually made between primary care (including GP services, and services provided by dentists and optometrists), secondary care (including standard hospital services), community care (including community nursing and a range of community-based services such as physiotherapy, occupational therapy and so on) and specialised care (including high-cost, low-volume services). Following the HSCA 2012, CCGs were responsible for commissioning secondary and community care, whilst

NHSE was responsible for primary and specialised care. In this book, references to primary care services predominantly mean primary medical care provided by GPs, as these are the services at which commissioning policy has been directed.

History of primary care commissioning and financing in England

The current primary care system in England is based on GPs being the contractors to the NHS rather than employees. This system was born out of the decision made at the establishment of the NHS in 1947 (Checkland et al, 2018b). This enabled GPs to remain independent of the NHS in a legal sense (although in reality the majority of practices depended overwhelmingly on NHS income), minimising their opposition to the NHS (Lewis, 1997; Peckham and Exworthy, 2003). From 1948 to 1990, there was little local planning and oversight of GP services, with GPs contracted as individuals and payment governed by the conditions set out and the number of patients registered with them. In 1990, a new GP contract was introduced known as the General Medical Services (GMS) contract. It sought to use contractual mechanisms to influence GP practice activity by introducing targets associated with payments for some services such as vaccinations and cervical smears. Prior to this contract, practices were paid for every vaccination and smear they provided; after the contract they only received payment if they met a pre-specified target. In addition the contract introduced payments for the provision of specific services.

In 2004, a newly negotiated national GMS contract was introduced combining a basic payment (calculated by a formula) with additional payment for meeting quality thresholds (known as the Quality and Outcomes Framework or QOF) and for providing a range of 'enhanced services'. There were three types of enhanced services:

1. Directed Enhanced Services (DES) – services provided by GP practices that have been negotiated nationally, such as extended opening hours;
2. National Enhanced Services (NES) – services commissioned from a GP practice using national specifications, such as minor injury services; and
3. Local Enhanced Services (LES) – locally developed services to meet local needs, such as services for asylum seekers and people with learning disabilities.

PCTs were tasked to develop schemes for local services to replace or supplement hospital services. PCTs were also given local flexibility using two additional contract types: personal medical services (PMS) and alternative providers of medical services (APMS). PMS contracts were to allow GPs to enter into a locally negotiated contract and be paid a fixed annual rate for provision of services negotiated with their PCT (Department of Health, 2003). In practice, PMS contracts, once negotiated, were not policed, and they tended to act to entrench income inequalities between practices (Majeed et al, 2012). APMS contracts were introduced to allow 'non-traditional' providers to encourage the setting up of new practices in 'under-doctored' areas (Department of Health, 2006b). In part, their use was intended to increase competitive pressures on traditional GP practices (Coleman et al, 2013).

Hence, since 1990, the NHS in England has combined local responsibility for planning with national responsibility for payment mechanisms and amounts. Local planners are only able to shift resources at the margins and room for local financial manoeuvre is limited, hence there are few levers to enact change. Local relationships and history of working together have become increasingly important (Best et al, 2012). Throughout the 2000s, various policies were introduced focusing on mechanisms to support local planning and quality improvement of primary care services. However, as negotiation of the base contract, which accounted for the majority of practice income, was constrained nationally, there remained limited freedom to shift resources around. Flexibilities focused on 'enhanced' services and procuring new practices via APMS contracts.

The reform following HSCA 2012 transferred the responsibilities for commissioning primary medical care services from PCTs to NHSE. Although CCGs would commission the majority of healthcare services, they would not be responsible for commissioning primary care services. This was to ensure a consistent and standardised national approach, as well as to alleviate concerns over conflicts of interest in terms of the possibility of GPs commissioning services that they themselves provided (Department of Health, 2010a).

Policy objectives

Since 2010, it was clear that to properly match primary care provision to the needs of an ageing population, local flexibility and understanding was required. There was considerable overlap between the 'core' GMS and PMS contracts (commissioned by NHSE) and services provided as 'enhanced services' (commissioned by CCGs). It seemed logical to bring those commissioning enhanced services into the process of commissioning the rest of primary care. Furthermore, the separation of funding streams between primary and community care meant that CCGs lacked the flexibility to shift funding to support patients most effectively at home.

In May 2014, following Simon Stevens' appointment as the Chief Executive of NHSE, CCGs were given 'new powers' to take on a greater role in commissioning primary care services. By delegating the primary care commissioning responsibilities from NHSE to CCGs (known as co-commissioning), CCGs would have greater power and influence over the commissioning of primary medical care which would enable them to take on a more integrated approach and 'unlock the full potential of their [CCGs'] statutory duty' (NHS England, 2014c, page 4). Although primary care services include medical, dental, eye health and pharmacy, the focus of the delegated responsibilities was on primary *medical* care.

It was claimed that the benefits of co-commissioning far outweigh the risks over conflicts of interests (NHS England, 2014c). CCGs would have more control of the wider NHS budget and this would enable a shift in investment from acute to primary and community services, improve access to primary care and out-of-hospital services, enable a more collaborative approach to designing local solutions for workforce and premises, and address challenges in information management and technology (NHS England, 2014a). In addition to better local services, co-commissioning would also enable the development of integrated out-of-hospital services and new models of care such as MCPs and PACSs, as set out in the FYFV (NHS England, 2014a).

The vision and aims of co-commissioning were described in relation to the wider agenda set out in the NHS FYFV (NHS England, 2014a):

> Co-commissioning is one of a series of changes set out in the NHS Five Year Forward View. The Forward View emphasises the need to increase the provision of out-of-hospital care and to break down barriers in how care is delivered. Co-commissioning is a key enabler in developing seamless, integrated out-of-hospital services based around the diverse needs of local populations. It will drive the development of new integrated out-of-hospital models of care, such as multispecialty community providers and primary and acute care systems ... Primary

care co-commissioning is the beginning of a longer journey towards place based commissioning. (NHS England, 2014a, page 11)

Hence the argument made in the HSCA 2012 for having primary care commissioning outside CCGs – that is, move towards a more standardised model of primary care commissioning – had shifted to an argument based upon the need to take into account different local contexts.

There are three co-commissioning models that CCGs could take forward: 'Greater involvement' – CCGs would have influence but not take the lead in shaping primary care locally; 'Joint commissioning' – CCGs would set up joint committees with NHSE regional teams to share primary care commissioning responsibility but funding would remain with NHSE finance so they remained party to all decision making; and 'Delegated authority' – CCGs would take on delegated responsibility of some aspect of primary care commissioning and take the lead on primary care commissioning. The scope of co-commissioning activities included designing, monitoring, negotiating and terminating core general medical services contracts (including GMS, PMS and APMS contracts) and newly designed enhanced services (LES and DES), designing local incentive schemes as an alternative to the QOF, making decisions on whether to establish new GP practices in an area, approving practice mergers and making decisions on 'discretionary' payments, for example, for premises reimbursement, returner/retainer schemes.

The policy was not without opposition, especially in terms of overcoming *real* and *perceived* conflicts associated with GPs commissioning or contracting themselves and performance management of the core GP contract of their members, with powers to issue breach notices and terminate contracts, as the key concerns. To mitigate worries over an increased risk of conflicts of interest, NHSE put in place a 'strengthened' approach and published statutory guidance on conflicts of interest (NHS England, 2014b, 2016a, 2017b). There was also uncertainty around what delegated responsibility actually involved and the voluntary nature of the arrangement (Royal College of General Practitioners and NHS Clinical Commissioners, 2014). CCGs had the option to 'do nothing' and not take up the options proposed. Although initially there was no clear expectation for all CCGs to move to delegated arrangements, in October 2015, one year following the policy implementation, NHSE 'encouraged' those CCGs still operating under 'joint commissioning' or 'greater involvement' to consider applying for full delegation by November 2015 (Dodge and Doyle, 2015). By 2016/17, 115 CCGs (out of 209) had moved towards delegated arrangements.

Study design and methods

The aim of the study was to understand the ways in which CCGs responded to their new primary care co-commissioning responsibilities from April 2015.

The study undertook an exploratory approach, combining data from interviews and national telephone surveys with analysis of policy documents and case studies. It adopted a realist evaluation approach in order to draw out programme theories motivating the policy of primary care co-commissioning. These programme theories were first elucidated during interviews with senior policy makers and were subsequently tested in the case studies.

Interviews with senior policy makers

The research started by carrying out a small number of face-to-face interviews ($n = 6$) with senior DH and NHSE staff (June to July 2015) who had played a role in the development of primary care co-commissioning policy. This was to understand the official aspirations and 'programme theories' (Weiss, 1997) underlying the policy. An in-depth analysis of the main policy documents related to co-commissioning was also undertaken.

CCG application documents

The uptake of primary care co-commissioning nationally (April to May 2015) was explored by reviewing CCGs' application documents as provided by NHSE with CCGs' agreement. A total of 147 applications from 150 CCGs were reviewed (some CCGs had submitted a joint application with their neighbouring CCGs and one CCG declined to take part). It was found that the amount of detail in each application varied widely, with some CCGs simply replicating what was in the official documents.

Telephone surveys

A sample of CCGs were selected to target for two telephone surveys (see Table 5.1). The first telephone survey was conducted at one

Table 5.1: Number of responses from telephone surveys

Levels	Number of CCGs taking over responsibility from April 15	Sample CCGs	Total response from the first survey	Total response from the second survey
Delegated	64	20	20	12
Joint	87	26	17	8
Greater involvement	58	58	12	1
TOTAL	209	104	49	21

year following the policy announcement (June to August 2015). The sampling criteria included; level of co-commissioning responsibility, regional team the CCG belonged to, size of CCG, urban versus rural CCG, those undertaking collaborative commissioning with neighbouring CCG or having submitted a joint application, and those adopting new models of care (NHS England, 2014a). The survey was repeated at two years following the policy announcement (August to October 2016). The same sample of CCGs was contacted. The second telephone survey was an opportunity to ask the initial sample of CCGs about the development of co-commissioning locally, to see whether their initial objectives for involvement were the same, whether the CCG had realised any benefits from the new responsibility and if they had made plans to move to a different level of co-commissioning. Between the first and second surveys, it was found that several people had left the organisation or changed job roles, which meant that recruitment was more problematic. Moreover, some of the interviewed CCGs had changed their level of responsibilities either from greater involvement to joint or delegated or from joint to delegated.

Case studies

Case studies were conducted in four CCGs nationally (January 2016 to April 2017). Table 5.2 outlines the site characteristics and data collected. Initially, the plan was to continue with two of the existing sites that had been involved in the CCG projects since 2010 (Checkland et al, 2012; McDermott et al, 2015; see also Chapters 3 and 4) and identify two new sites based on findings from the first telephone survey. However, it was found that even those sites that had previously been involved with the research were quite reluctant take part. Once access to sites had

Table 5.2: Site characteristics and data collection

	Site 1	Site 2	Site 3	Site 4
Region	North	Midlands & East	South	North
Level	Delegated	Delegated	Delegated	Initially joint but have moved to delegated
Population	Over 40 practices with population approx. 350K	Over 100 practices with population approx. 550K	Over 20 practices with population approx. 150K	Over 40 practices with population approx. 250K
Contract	Majority PMS practices, some GMS and APMS	All practices switched from PMS to GMS, no APMS	Majority GMS practices, some PMS and no APMS	Almost equal number of PMS and GMS practices, some APMS
Vanguard	Yes	Yes	None	None
Federation	Yes	Yes	None	Yes
Sustainability & Transformation Plan (STP)	STP1	STP2	STP3	STP1
Number of meetings attended	13	24	6	31
Number of interviews conducted	7	13	11	11

been agreed, there was also some difficulty in accessing a full range of meetings, with some sites reluctant to allow attendance at non-public meetings. Concerns included issues of confidentiality and concerns about sharing of commercially sensitive information.

Observations focused mainly on meetings associated with primary care co-commissioning. These included the Primary Care Commissioning Committee (PCCC) and its subcommittees or subgroups with such names as strategy committee, operational committee and quality committee. A total of 74 meetings (approximately 111 hours of observations) were attended; and a total of 42 face-to-face interviews were conducted with members of the PCCC, such as the Lay Chair, Primary Care Manager, Head of Contract, Head of Quality, Head of Estates, Head of Engagement, Local Medical Council representative, and Director of Healthwatch. The CCGs' GB Chair, Accountable Officer, and Chief Finance Officer were also interviewed.

Programme theory versus the practice of co-commissioning

The problems identified in documents and interviews and the suggested solutions are outlined in Figure 5.1. The suggested solutions fed into the development of two programme theories underpinning the decision to delegate primary care commissioning responsibilities from NHSE to CCGs.

Theory 1

Theory 1 concerned the integration of budgets and commissioning responsibility with a single commissioner for commissioning primary, community and secondary care for a geographical population. This would allow the shifting of resources between sectors, facilitate the development of a more integrated approach to service provision, and provide an environment that would support the development of integrated organisations delivering new models of care as envisaged in the FYFV (NHS England, 2014a). This would then deliver more care outside hospitals, and care which, from the patient's perspective, is more integrated and would be more efficient, effective and cheaper.

Theory 2

Theory 2 was that CCGs understood primary care and local needs. Allowing CCGs to commission primary care alongside other services the CCG was already commissioning would support the development and implementation of local strategies for service improvement, support innovation in primary care, and allow investment in primary care (by allowing resource shifting as previously discussed). This would improve quality of care, make primary care a more attractive place to work, and facilitate GP recruitment and retention.

In practice, it was found that Theory 2 provided a better description of how CCGs viewed the process (for more detail see McDermott et al, 2016b). The CCGs surveyed said that their main objectives for taking on co-commissioning responsibility were to enable them to commission primary care alongside the commissioning of other services, which was seen as an important gap caused by the HSCA 2012. This would give them an opportunity for local decision making

Figure 5.1: Problems identified in documents and interviews – and suggested solutions

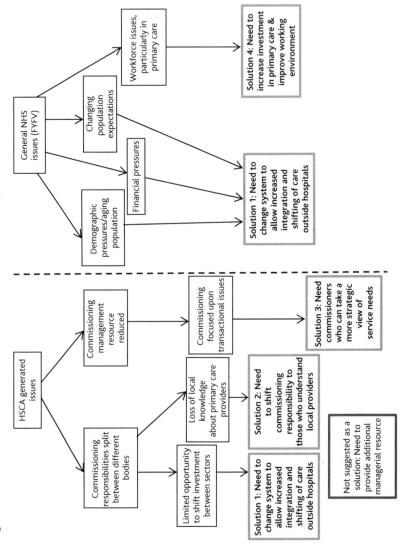

and local flexibility and allow them to improve investment in primary care and increase quality.

There was little mention of place-based commissioning, new models of care, or an outcome-based approach, despite these being much discussed in policy documents and interviews with senior policy makers. This suggested that immediate concerns of CCGs revolved around the need to ensure sustainable high-quality primary care services, but that some were aware of the longer-term potential to start to think creatively about how services were provided across a local geography. There was a local aim of trying to 'piece commissioning back together', which in turn would encourage integration and wider transformation work. The ability to commission a whole pathway, from primary care to secondary care, was perceived as a mechanism to improve the quality of services. Overall, as membership organisations, co-commissioning responsibility was seen by CCGs as an opportunity to support primary care, redesign services and improve the relationship with the CCG membership.

Two years following the policy implementation, when the second telephone survey was conducted, it was found that the initial objectives for CCGs' involvement in the commissioning of primary care had remained the same for both joint and delegated commissioning. Local flexibility and influence were still perceived to be the main benefits of the new commissioning arrangements; some CCGs believed that the new responsibility would provide a step towards more place-based commissioning and in some cases the formation of ACOs. The level of primary care commissioning responsibility was found to impact on the achievements and outcomes that were discussed by CCG staff.

Results

Co-commissioning activity

Findings from the case study CCGs showed that they were largely focusing their efforts in three areas: (1) reactive work required to manage ongoing issues, including legacy issues inherited from NHSE which involved estates or issues to do with APMS contracts; (2) proactive development of primary care strategies and plans (including development of 'new' incentive schemes); and (3) a national scheme to improve estates and information systems.

Primary care strategies were largely focused upon: improving the quality of care provided; encouraging practices to work together in larger groups to provide standardised access and/or a more integrated approach to delivering health and social care services; and developing general practice 'at scale' to enable greater delivery of out-of-hospital services and delivery of care closer to home. The mechanism to bring about these changes focused upon financial incentivisation of areas of work such as: commitment to a range of care standards, including proactive care of vulnerable patients; improved access; development of co-operative working between practices to deliver a wider range of services, including the formation of formal federations; and medicines management and prescribing. These schemes were funded via the existing primary care budget (with the reinvestment of funds previously used to support PMS contracts), consolidation of existing DES and LES, and the wider CCG budget (although this was limited by budgetary pressures, with some CCGs forced to use primary care funds to support secondary care budgets). The focus on estates and technology was driven by a national funding scheme.

These approaches and strategies bear a strong resemblance to incentive schemes developed under the PBC initiative which preceded the HSCA 2012 (Checkland et al, 2009; Coleman et al, 2010; see also Chapter 4).

Comparison with Practice-Based Commissioning (PBC)

The study revealed many similarities between the work undertaken by CCGs under co-commissioning and the work previously undertaken under PBC. The most obvious difference between the two was that CCGs undertaking primary care co-commissioning also carried responsibility for GMS, PMS and APMS contracts. Work to harmonise (that is, reduce funding differentials) between PMS and GMS practices began under the auspices of PCTs, was continued by NHSE and then fell to CCGs to complete. The money freed up by the equalisation of funding formed a large part of the investment fund that CCGs used to support their various incentive and 'add on contract' schemes. In addition, CCGS were responsible for making decisions about APMS contracts. This latter work was complicated by: the need to avoid conflicts of interest, which limited the ability of local GPs to contribute; the fact that some CCGs lacked the required expertise with respect to estates and contract management; and some confusion over what was or was not done by NHSE with respect to these contracts. However, the core GMS contract remained nationally negotiated, and little enthusiasm was observed in the case study CCGs for changing its basic provisions. Even those CCGs involved in the Vanguard programme focused their efforts in primary care around additional 'contracts' rather than making changes to the core contract.

Those involved with primary care co-commissioning were asked to reflect upon the similarities with PBC which had been observed. The differences that were highlighted were differences in tone and scale, rather than in direction of travel or focus.

> 'The fundamental ... the biggest difference is we've got more GPs seeing a bigger picture and being more strategic if you like. PBC was about small-scale, little pet projects about half a whole time physiotherapist in a couple of practices or a bit of a path ... a bunion pathway or a ... You know? [...] PBC was not about big transformational change, it was about ... it was almost GP fundholding. You know it was GPs who saw that it was about their business.' (Manager ID12)

> 'And I just think co-commissioning is a reinvention of practice-based commissioning, to be fair. But it needs to be under a different guise. The NHS is always reinventing themselves, but they call it something different. But historically they go round in circles, and end up where they have come from. I think that's what is co-commissioning, to be fair.' (NHSE representative ID48)

This is an important observation, as it highlights the fact that, whilst the establishment of CCGs was intended to overcome the perceived weaknesses of the PBC programme, in practice it failed to engage with the realities of PBC in many areas. In particular, many PBC groups had most success in developing collective provision of primary care-based services (Coleman et al, 2009), but CCGs were precluded from commissioning such services. The introduction of primary care co-commissioning was used by many CCGs to allow them to reintroduce such schemes, raising important questions about the loss of momentum associated with the HSCA 2012.

Conflicts of interest

Conflicts of interest took on increased importance when co-commissioning put GPs in the position of both commissioners and providers of primary care. In December 2014, NHSE published statutory guidance on how CCGs should manage conflicts of interest (NHS England, 2014b) in recognition that co-commissioning would expose CCGs to a greater risk of both *real* and *perceived* conflicts of interest. Following that, the guidance has been strengthened through various revisions (NHS England, 2016a, 2017b). CCGs had to verify that they had plans in place to comply with the guidance when they applied to take on delegated or joint commissioning responsibilities, as well as during the annual CCG performance-assessment process.

The risk of conflicts of interest arises from the public stewardship role that GPs assume in their position of commissioners of primary care (Moran et al, 2017a). This differs fundamentally from their role as private providers contracted by the NHS to deliver primary care services. Respondents stated that they perceived the risk of conflicts of interest concerning processes such as: obtaining clinical input for contract and service specifications; supporting the development of GP provider organisations; GPs' influence over discussions and decision making; and GPs' perceived bias towards the provision of services by GP practices. Thus, a central issue was the public interest and ensuring value for money for public funds. It was regarded as necessary for GPs, as the custodians of public funds, to persuade the public that the CCG had no vested interests. The *perception* of a conflict of interest was viewed as being just as serious as an actual conflict of interest.

Two types of conflicts of interest that arose from CCGs taking on co-commissioning were identified. One was GPs' influence over discussions and decision making as well as GPs' potential bias towards primary care. The other was from committee members other than GPs and practice managers, including lay members. Although GPs were in the minority on the PCCC, they could unduly influence decisions and this more ambiguous conflict of interest was more difficult to deal with than more overt conflict of interest. GPs had 'soft power', in terms of being able to exert authority and influence over decision making rather than relying on hierarchical supervision or sanctions (Courpasson, 2000). To mitigate this, GPs in the case study sites who declared a conflict of interest were asked to either leave the room or stay in the room but not participate in the discussion and vote. However, there was a lack of consistency in this practice both within and between CCGs, meaning that GPs were sometimes involved in discussions about funding and contracts. The 'soft' influence was less apparent when the CCG employed an independent GP, which implied that GPs' pre-existing relationships with other committee members may be important.

There was some cognisance that the GP membership were not always happy with the new policy. GPs on the GB felt divorced from the PCCC and this caused frustration as primary care was their area of expertise and the separation could inhibit a strategic overview of the CCGs' responsibilities:

> 'It leaves GP leaders like me frustrated because some of the conflicts of interest and governance means that I don't get to see a full picture that I like, because as a strategist, and responsible for the vision of where we're going, I need to understand a broad brush of everything.' (CCG Chair GP ID8)

Moreover, asking GPs to leave the room could lead to a situation in which a group of people (lay members and executive managers) had to make clinically related decisions without any clinical input. This highlighted a contradiction which sits at the heart of the CCG model – CCGs being GP-led organisations having to reduce or remove clinical involvement from primary care commissioning decisions due to concerns over conflicts of interest.

There was resentment that while GPs did not create the issue of conflicts of interest, they were seemingly blamed for it. However, it was felt that the procedures were necessary, even if they were not always popular. GPs' conflicts were an inevitable consequence of them being knowledgeable about their subject and possessing the local knowledge cited as a benefit of having GPs commissioning primary care. Hence, conflicts of interest are something to be managed rather than eliminated and CCGs had to perform a balancing act between utilising the important input of GPs in terms of knowledge of local health issues and the conflicts that stemmed from GPs as members of the organisation holding their contracts.

Locally based primary care plans versus wider national initiatives

The case study CCGs suggested that, unrelated to primary care commissioning, changes to the organisations and demands placed on them from the national level had caused the CCGs' relationship with their members to deteriorate. The need to implement national policy often made the membership feel that they were not part of the decision-making process and there was concern that some would feel disenfranchised by this. The case study CCGs tried to manage the demands that were placed upon them by NHSE (central policy) whilst fostering a sense of membership on a local footprint with their member practices. This proved to be a challenge for the CCGs.

Although many members embraced national policy in response to the CCG implementing the objectives of the FYFV (NHS England, 2014a), there were tensions from others who did not understand either the CCGs' role in co-commissioning or the need to move towards collaborative general practice.

As primary care was seen as something to be planned and commissioned locally, there were concerns about how this local plan would align with the wider national initiatives. Respondents likened this process to a 'jigsaw'. One of the challenges for CCGs was to keep the connectivity between the two. However, this would require additional work and would increase the pressure on already stretched resources.

The case study CCGs described how they needed to grapple with understanding which services could be planned and commissioned locally, on a 'place' basis, and which could be provided on a 'wider footprint'. The deliberation seems to be around population size, geographical footprint, relationship with local hospitals and LA, and the current system in place. Another respondent said that one of the factors affecting the discussion about service provision on a 'wider footprint' was to do with the level of specialism and expertise required in delivering that service.

It was unclear to the case study CCGs how wider national initiatives could drive and support primary care, which is very much about locality. There was also incongruence between the CCGs, national policy and the democratic processes of what it means to be a membership organisation. This was found to impact on both the CCGs and their members in most sites, who described similar issues in feeling frustration over their responsibilities to NHSE and contradictions of 'having to' enact policy rather than collectively discuss and act in the interest of local needs. In addition to national policy, national targets on which CCGs were monitored were found in some instances to cause tension and disengagement with the GPs.

The sense of disconnect between local needs and regional/national-level decision making, added to concern that integration between health and social care would erode the clinical leadership which is inherent in CCGs, led to a growing disenfranchisement amongst GP members in the case study CCGs.

Unintended consequences

In exercising the co-commissioning responsibilities, CCGs were required to establish a PCCC, which is a decision-making committee. CCGs were given the flexibility to articulate each PCCC's responsibilities, its membership, quorum, schedules, frequency of meetings, accountability, procurement and decision making. The initial guidance only stipulated that the committee must have a lay and executive majority and have a lay chair (NHS England, 2014c). While this leaves room for local specificity in the process of shaping the governance structure, it also led to varying degrees of ambiguity in relation to what was expected from CCGs, or how best to define responsibilities, domains of operation, and lines of accountability. As was found in the early part of the longitudinal study following the development of CCGs (Checkland et al, 2016; also see Chapter 3), this flexibility led to considerable variation in the makeup of committees. There was a line of reporting from PCCC to the CCG GB, but the PCCC was set up as independent of the GB. Respondents in the case studies identified the PCCC as a 'sort of governing body for primary care' or as 'sitting beside the governing body'. This caused concern in some CCGs over a possibility of the PCCC having an equal power to the GB.

As NHSE still held the statutory responsibility, early in the process there was some confusion around whether certain functions could be legally delegated to CCGs, for example, complaints management. In the initial guidance it was stated that delegated CCGs would be responsible for complaints management (NHS England, 2014c). However, NHSE later clarified that 'under the current legal framework NHSE cannot delegate complaints management to CCGs, although a management arrangement could be implemented' (NHS England, 2015b). Another example was freedom of information requests, as they covered both organisations. There was also an issue with 'double delegation'. Several CCGs said that they had initially planned to form joint committees with neighbouring CCGs. In one of the CCGs, their application was signed off by NHSE before their own legal team advised them that it was a 'double delegation', which was not legally permitted (McDermott et al, 2016b). This led to some CCGs restructuring their governance arrangements.

The ramification of the HSCA 2012, and particularly the abolition of PCTs, was felt strongly in the domain of property management as legislation proved very unclear. Primary care estate is a complex area, with a complicated patchwork of property ownership, including ownership by individuals, ownership by partnerships, standard leasing arrangements and private finance initiative leases. A main and persistent issue was the problem of nominating a head lease for buildings and how current contractual designs posed challenges. While CCGs were expected to devise local strategies, which often included estate development, practice mergers, or expansion – especially in light of policy climates that favoured commissioning 'at scale' (see Chapter 3) – they still lacked the legal framework with which to mandate such changes and operationalise their estate programmes.

Discussion

Primary care co-commissioning is a relatively new approach, and there is little published research. NHSE produced a number of 'case studies' which set out the benefits of delegated responsibility for primary care co-commissioning (NHS England, 2017a)

These were intended to encourage CCGs that did not undertake full delegated responsibility to move to full delegation; they were therefore focused upon the positive aspects of the transition. The claimed benefits fell into three main categories: service improvements arising out of CCG plans or strategies; benefits arising out of the closer relationship between the CCG and member practices necessary to commission primary care services; and longer-term potential benefits associated with clinical involvement in commissioning primary care. These claims to benefit depend upon the baseline being used. If the comparison is with primary care commissioning undertaken by NHSE, then it is clear that the greater local knowledge and understanding of CCGs is important in ensuring that primary care services meet local needs, and the findings are consistent with this. The study also found some evidence to support the claim that GP practices, as CCG members, had become more engaged with their CCG as a result. In particular, the opportunity to tailor additional contract/incentive schemes to meet local needs was valuable in engaging practices and supporting change. However, the comparison with PBC on pages 74–75 suggested that the improvement to services was qualitatively similar to that which was being pursued by PCTs under the PBC initiative.

Research by the King's Fund and the Nuffield Trust explored the engagement of GPs with their local CCG. The most recent findings from this study (Robertson et al, 2015) suggested that GPs were supportive of their CCG taking over responsibility for commissioning primary care, and were happy for the CCG to have a role in improving the quality of care provided. However, they were less happy with the CCG having a more formal performance management role and were keen for primary care commissioning to be led by local clinicians. This latter point highlighted the issues with endemic conflicts of interest which have been explored: clinical leadership brings with it inevitable conflicts of interest.

Research has suggested that GP engagement with commissioning via the PBC initiative was feasible and could potentially add significant value, but its practice was dependent to a large degree, on the attitude and approach of the host PCT (Miller et al, 2015; also see Chapter 4). An appetite was found amongst GPs for peer review of performance, and there was evidence of increasing attempts to improve the quality and range of services provided in the community, although little sign of wider impact on commissioning of secondary care services. Other studies have highlighted the variable nature of engagement by GPs and practices (Curry and Thorlby, 2007), a finding mirrored by the King's Fund/Nuffield study of CCGs (Robertson et al, 2016). A report published in 2010 highlighted the need to consider the scale at which particular types of services needed to be commissioned, with a focus upon setting up structures which would allow pooling of resources between commissioning bodies in order to commission secondary care services which required a significant population base, whilst retaining local responsiveness for primary care and other community-based services (Smith et al, 2010). That has resonance with this study, which highlighted the perceived importance of local involvement in primary care commissioning.

The study showed that the commissioning of primary care required detailed local knowledge about services and providers alongside expertise in the unique domain of primary care, and that primary care co-commissioning by CCGs had the potential to provide this more effectively than was the case when NHSE retained full responsibility for primary care commissioning. It is likely that the potential for these benefits to be realised will depend crucially upon the provision of sufficient managerial expertise. In addition, primary care co-commissioning by CCGs carries within it the potential for investment that will break down barriers between primary, secondary and community services. However, it is too early for this to have been realised. The involvement of GPs in the commissioning of primary care services is regarded as positive, both in terms of engaging local GPs and in ensuring that new services meet local needs. However, conflicts of interest are inherent to this process, and will require ongoing management.

The current legislative framework within which CCGs are taking on their additional responsibilities is not fit for purpose. The fact that NHSE retains statutory responsibility for primary care commissioning fundamentally limits the ability of CCGs to act in some areas. The evidence suggests that primary care co-commissioning by CCGs is likely to more effectively support the development of primary care services than would be the case had NHSE retained the responsibility.

However, comparison with PBC also shows that what is happening under primary care co-commissioning does not differ in fundamental ways from the work that was being undertaken by PCTs via the PBC initiative prior to the HSCA 2012. This similarity suggests that the approach being adopted – local development of plans alongside strategic use of funding to incentivise desired behaviours by GP practices – is the approach most suited to the current contractual landscape of general practice. Current broader policy initiatives such as the Vanguard programme suggest an appetite amongst policy makers to change this contractual landscape (NHS England, 2014a), but the study has not found a significant appetite amongst GPs for this.

In summary, the study showed that CCGs were generally enthusiastic about the opportunity to take greater responsibility in this area and had aspirations to develop more integrated services for patients. Over time, most CCGs have moved to take on full delegated responsibility for commissioning GP services, and have established functioning PCCCs, with little evidence of significant problems associated with conflicts of interest. However, conflicts of interest are inherent to this process, and will require ongoing management. The commissioning of primary care requires detailed local knowledge about services and providers alongside expertise in the unique domain of primary care, and delegated responsibilities have the potential to provide this more effectively than was the case when NHSE retained full responsibility for primary care commissioning. It is likely that the potential for these benefits to be realised will require the contextual condition of sufficient managerial expertise. In addition, primary care co-commissioning by CCGs carries within it the potential for investment that will break down barriers between primary, secondary and community service. However, it is as yet too early for this to have been realised. Furthermore, no appetite was found for fundamental changes to GP core contracts, and it is likely that such investment will take place via 'add-on contracts' or incentive schemes. The involvement of GPs in the commissioning of primary care services is regarded as positive, both in terms of engaging local GPs and in ensuring that new services meet local needs. There have been significant local legacy issues in some areas relating to unclear contracts and poor handover of responsibilities from NHSE. The current legislation, under which statutory responsibility for commissioning primary care services remains with NHSE and is delegated rather than transferred to CCGs, presents some problems, particularly for those CCGs that wish to work together across a broader geographical footprint.

6

Commissioning of healthcare through competitive and cooperative mechanisms under the HSCA 2012

Dorota Osipovic, Pauline Allen, Elizabeth Shepherd, Christina Petsoulas, Anna Coleman, Neil Perkins, Lorraine Williams and Marie Sanderson

Introduction

Competition and cooperation are the two fundamental mechanisms of service procurement in the NHS and represent the tools for 'getting things done'. This chapter presents empirical findings from a longitudinal, qualitative case study research project into the use of competition and cooperation by local NHS commissioners following the HSCA 2012.

As outlined in Chapter 2, the economics of markets (and their opposite, hierarchies) in conjunction with more sophisticated theories of cooperation underpin the analysis of competition and cooperation in the NHS quasi-market. For a market to operate competitively, there needs to be sufficient numbers of buyers and sellers of goods and services. A key assumption is that purchasers have sufficient information about the goods or services to make rational choices and maximise their utility. The market will produce value for money by allocating resources to the best use at the most efficient price (Allen, 2013).

Competition in the NHS is realised through several models. Competition *for* the market is a result of tendering processes whereby different providers compete to deliver a particular service and one provider wins the whole market. Competition *within* the market exists when a number of providers are accredited to provide a particular service and they compete to attract patients. An example of the competition *for* the market is tendering out of community health services, and an example of competition *within* the market is the patient choice of elective secondary or community-based care.

In order to analyse cooperation the theory of 'co-opetition' and the work of Elinor Ostrom (2005) are utilised. Co-opetition suggests that organisations can compete and cooperate simultaneously to mutual benefit (Brandenburger and Nalebuff, 1996). Ostrom suggests that individuals can self-organise to solve collective problems, without direct control by the government, and can establish and enforce rules limiting the appropriation of common pool resources.

In terms of defining cooperation, there are a number of closely related terms such as collaboration, coordination, integrated care, networking and partnership. Integrated care implies the coordination of separate but interconnected components which should function together to perform a shared task (Kodner and Spreeuwenberg, 2002). Cooperation can take place at a service, organisational or clinical level (Fulop et al, 2005). It can occur horizontally between providers of similar services, or vertically between different sectors (for example, primary and secondary care). Cooperation between different organisations may involve sharing of the resources, risks, know-how, strategic information or new markets whilst working towards mutually beneficial goals. Partners need to have a shared understanding of policy and rules for such a partnership to be successful.

Commissioners have the dual objective of promoting cooperation between different providers in terms of clinical service delivery and fostering cooperation between providers and commissioners themselves for the purposes of strategic planning and ongoing monitoring of service provision.

While studies have noted that incentives for competition and cooperation exist in healthcare, few have researched the interaction between the two (Goddard and Mannion, 1998; Kurunmaki, 1999). Some studies also dealt with particular aspects of competition or cooperation. For instance, Krachler and Greer (2015) undertook a study of the relationship between marketisation and privatisation in the post-HSCA 2012 NHS. The study focused on market entry by private providers. Some specific forms of cooperation have also been evaluated, such as integrated care (Erens et al, 2016; RAND Europe and Ernst and Young, 2012) and clinical networks, but the manner in which local health systems were being managed to balance competition and cooperation under the HSCA 2012 has not been investigated.

When the HSCA 2012 came into force there was lack of clarity as to what these legislative changes meant for services on the ground. It has been pointed out that the provisions of the HSCA 2012 concerning competition were hard to follow and might be inconsistent (Hazell, 2014). Given the lack of clarity around the rules and the simultaneous requirements to follow both competition and cooperation enshrined in the legislation, it was important to investigate how commissioners on the ground understood and applied the regulations of HSCA 2012 and interpreted national policy signals.

There were a number of ways of coping with the ambiguity inherent in the commissioning policy landscape. For instance, a popular method of procurement which has developed under the auspices of the guidance from NHS national bodies since 2013 was that of 'Most Capable Provider' (MCProv), under which commissioners used a transparent process to identify the best provider but did not continue with a full formal competitive procurement process once this provider had been chosen. According to Mills & Reeve (2016), 'MCProv' is an unofficial expression, which was used by commissioners and has been approved by Monitor (the predecessor to NHSI) as a process compliant with the 2013 Procurement Regulations. It refers either to: (a) a competitive process (generally featuring dialogue or negotiation) involving the selection of potential providers from a limited pool who were either identified by the commissioner as being possible suppliers following a research or consultation exercise, or who might have responded to an advertisement or engagement event (but possibly with a limited geographic reach) and were therefore interested in participating; or (b) a negotiated procedure with a single provider identified by the commissioner as obviously being the most capable of providing a particular service in a particular locality.

A new set of pro-competitive regulations with statutory effect came into force in respect of the NHS in April 2016: the Public Contract Regulations 2015 (PCR 2015). Application of the PCR 2015 to commissioning NHS services has been interpreted as having introduced a requirement to advertise in the *Official Journal of the European Union* (OJEU) any contract for health services whose value exceeds a stipulated threshold (Mills & Reeve, 2016). However, the prevailing view was that there was no requirement to follow a full competitive procurement. As a result, this process has been labelled a 'Light Touch Regime' (Crown Commercial Service, 2016; Mills & Reeve, 2016). This view has been supported by the Department of Health (2016), the regulator, NHSI (NHSI, 2016) and NHSE (NHSE, 2016).

There were a number of regulatory decisions, as well as speeches and statements by influential policy makers, which indicated a shift towards cooperative coordination in the commissioning of healthcare services in England. A particularly salient regulatory decision was news that the two NHS FTs in Bournemouth and Poole, which were prohibited from merging by the national competition regulator in 2013 (Competition Commission, 2013; Sanderson et al, 2017) could merge after all (Carding, 2017). Furthermore, on several occasions Simon Stevens (Chief Executive Officer of NHSE) stated that competition was not appropriate for NHS organisations, which needed to reduce their 'institutional self-interest' in the interests of the whole local health economy (eg Dunhill, 2016; Thomas and West, 2017).

The changes in the national policy on commissioning mechanisms were not accompanied by the corresponding changes in the legislation, with all provisions of the HSCA 2012 remaining in force. This created a space for a disjuncture between regulation and practice of commissioning. Ultimately, it was the role of NHS commissioners, including local CCGs led by GPs, to ensure the appropriate levels of competition and cooperation in their local health economies.

Study design and methods

In light of the absence of evidence about the operation of the competition aspects of the HSCA 2012 from the viewpoint of CCG commissioners, a study was undertaken to investigate how commissioners in local health systems managed the interplay of competition and cooperation in their local health economies, looking at acute, mental health and community health services. The research questions were:

- How do commissioners and the organisations they commission from understand the policy and regulatory environment, including incentives for competition and cooperation?
- In the environment which encourages both competition and cooperation, how do commissioning organisations and providers approach their relationships with each other in order to undertake the planning and delivery of care for patients?
- How do commissioning organisations use or shape the local provider environment to secure high-quality care for patients?

In order to answer the research questions a qualitative, longitudinal case study research design was adopted, looking in depth at four CCG areas in England. The case study sites comprised a mix of rural and urban settings and were located in the North, the Midlands and London.

Table 6.1: Interviews by case study site and wave

Case study site	Location of CCG	Wave 1	Wave 2	Wave 3	Total
CCG1	Rural, North	10	2	3	15
CCG2	Urban, Midlands	9	2	4	15
CCG3	Mixed, North	7	2	3	12
CCG4	London	7	3	5	15
Total		33	9	15	57

Table 6.2: Interviews by case study site, type of provider and service

			CCG1	CCG2	CCG3	CCG4	Total
Commissioners			9	7	4	6	26
Providers	NHS	Acute	3	1	2	4	10
		CHS and/ or MH	2	5	4	3	14
	Non-NHS	CHS and/ or MH	1	2	2	2	7
Total			15	15	12	15	57

Case study sites were selected in order to reflect the diversity of local populations and different configurations of local providers. The use of case studies was deemed the most appropriate research design as case studies allow for exploration of mechanisms, processes and phenomena in real-life contexts (Yin, 2009).

The study consisted of three waves of interviews with commissioners and providers in four case study sites conducted over a period of four years, 2013–17. A total of 57 interviews were conducted (see Table 6.1).

The interviewed commissioner and provider managers were senior level managers at chief executive or director level, mostly with no clinical background. The interviewed providers represented the key acute, community and mental health services providers of a particular CCG and comprised both NHS and independent sector organisations (see Table 6.2). The same set of organisations (and the same interviewees, where possible) were followed during the successive waves.

Throughout the study local documents such as CCG GB papers and procurement portals were also consulted to gather information on commissioning strategies, financial status and use of competitive tendering in each of the four CCGs. Some of the findings from various stages of the study have been reported elsewhere (Allen et al, 2014a,

2016, 2017; Osipovic et al, 2016, 2017; Sanderson et al, 2017). This chapter offers a summary of the findings.

The first part of this chapter focuses on outlining the views of commissioners and providers on the regulatory landscape, in particular their understanding of regulations prior to and after the publication of the FYFV in October 2014, which marked an important policy change. The second part explores commissioners' use of competition and cooperation commissioning mechanisms and providers' experiences of competition and cooperation.

Findings

Understanding and experience of the regulatory framework under HSCA 2012

As actors' understandings of the rules under which they operate are crucial in determining their behaviour, participants were asked about their understanding of policy, guidance and the regulatory framework regarding the use of competition and cooperation in commissioning NHS services. In the case of the English NHS these rules consist of both legislation (primary – that is, acts of parliament; and secondary – that is, statutory instruments) and policies issued by the DH and NHSE.

Commissioners in each site considered the HSCA 2012 confusing as they were expected to both drive competition and integrate services, which they found to be contradictory: "Those two drivers can compete against each other" (Commissioner 3, CCG4, May 2014). Some commissioners were awaiting guidance on how to implement policy, or commented that where there was guidance, interpretation was likened to "trawling through treacle" (Commissioner 1, CCG1, May 2014).

When asked about their understanding regarding whether the current policies required them to tender all services, commissioners were convinced that this was not the case. There was a consensus that although there was no mandate to tender all services, there was a requirement to justify the occasions when competitive procurement was not pursued.

Lack of explicit, unambiguous guidance about the role of competition in commissioning clinical services could in some cases play to commissioners' advantage by increasing their freedom. However, it also increased the freedom of providers to challenge commissioning decisions and/or to interpret the regulatory uncertainty to their advantage. A commissioner from CCG1 cited a case of a private provider offering maternity services in the region and expecting to be paid by the local CCGs despite not being commissioned by them. Such provider behaviour, driven by patient choice and effectively bypassing commissioners, undermined the level of control commissioners had over their local health economies.

Provider managers were also confused about the meaning of the competition rules. They echoed commissioners' concerns about the vagueness and complexity of the formal rules and a need for better guidance.

The lack of sufficiently specific guidance about the HSCA 2012 resulted in commissioners having to consult sector regulators. Commissioners were often quite critical of the role of sector regulators, mainly due to their alleged inability to provide clear guidance in particular cases.

In common with commissioners, the regulation of the health sector was seen as muddled by provider managers, with Monitor having conflicting duties. One felt that the relationship between the different regulators was not clear and there was no overall organisation responsible for regulation: "The interactions between the different regulators is confused. [...] There used to be ... an organisation that was clearly responsible for ... holding the ring, in the shape of SHAs [Strategic Health Authorities], that's disappeared" (Provider 2, NHS, acute, CCG2, March 2014).

Changes in understanding of the regulatory framework after the publication of the five year forward view

Commissioners in all the case study sites, who were re-interviewed in 2015, after the publication of the FYFV, noted a change in tone of national policy messages towards greater promotion of collaboration in commissioning. They thought that the FYFV legitimised local cooperative initiatives aiming to transform services and it allowed them greater latitude in deciding whether to tender out services. However, at the same time, commissioners pointed out that none of the underlying rules guiding procurement of clinical services had changed as a result of the FYFV and warned that the rules could not be disregarded completely.

The different national bodies, some in favour of cooperation (NHS England) and some still promoting the use of competition (Monitor), were sending conflicting messages. Despite a reduction in its use, most of the re-interviewed commissioners saw a need for competition to remain available to them as a commissioning tool to use at their discretion.

The policy push towards collaborative commissioning was even more discernible in the interviews conducted in 2017. Despite the pro-competitive rules laid out in the HSCA 2012 and the PCR 2015, both national policy and commissioning reality on the ground were found to have changed substantially, turning in favour of the use of the cooperative mechanisms and organisational solutions which put competition "on the backburner" (Provider 1, NHS, CHS and/or MH, CCG3, June 2017).

> 'I think [the rules] are unchanged really, if I'm honest. I think the context is changed and I think the political imperatives around this are changing, so it feels to me increasingly that the NHS is unhappy with the concept of the internal market and PbR and contracting and everything else, and is focusing or trying to focus much more on collaboration and partnership and, you know, work through STPs and that kind of approach.' (Commissioner 1, CCG2, June 2017)

Participants also moved on from the preoccupation with a lack of clarity in the existing rules, noted during the first wave of the fieldwork. Instead they stressed that the existing rules did not sufficiently support the national policy direction towards cooperation. Since the introduction of STPs and ACOs/ACSs, local commissioners and providers were being asked to come together in search of locally agreed solutions to address various service delivery pressures in the context of deteriorating financial resources. The energy of commissioners and providers was directed towards searching for such solutions, rather than on the interpretation of rules.

Despite acknowledging (and in many cases embracing) the turn to cooperation, commissioner and provider managers interviewed in 2017 could not ignore the rules entirely, partly for fear of legal challenge and partly as the sector regulators still appraised the financial and clinical performance of their organisations separately. The regulatory system set up to uphold and enforce the rules of the internal market in healthcare was still in place.

Some commissioners noted that the disjuncture between the rules and policy could become a stumbling block on the road to STP and ACO implementation. In particular, it was not clear to some commissioners and providers whether the new models of care and budding ACOs could be commissioned outside of the competitive procurement framework. Commissioners and providers closely observed developing practices in this respect.

The independent providers interviewed in 2017 were generally wary of the policy turn to collaboration, but at the same time saw some opportunities that came with it in terms of collaborative engagement with other providers. The independent providers wanted to see a more robust enforcement of the rules enabling competition within the healthcare sector.

Use and experience of competition and cooperative mechanisms under HSCA 2012

In order to understand how competition and cooperation were used locally in the case study sites, the major service delivery issues were investigated, to determine how they were approached.

The urgent need to find savings had been made clear by NHSE in July 2013, and dominated local agendas. Each case study site was engaged in efforts to move care out of hospital into the community, in the hope that money would be saved.

In order to tackle these big service reconfiguration challenges, the four CCGs were generally exploring collaborative approaches. Commissioners on the whole took the route of coordinating cooperation between themselves and providers. They did not use competitive processes to make major changes. The complexity of the issues involved in such reconfigurations required an iterative approach using a series of meetings with local providers at which actors were encouraged to come to a collective agreement about how changes would be made.

Commissioners in all sites were exploring the option of using outcome-based commissioning approaches as well as lead provider models for a range of different services (see Chapter 7). In two sites – CCG4 and CCG1 – the outcome-based commissioning approach was going to be used to redesign the provision of CHS. Commissioners hoped that prime provider models and outcome-based contracts would remove cost pressures associated with the "open chequebook" (Commissioner 3, CCG1, April 2014) pricing structure of PbR by moving to capitated budgets. Although these approaches could have involved competitive tendering, they did not do so in the case study sites. Instead, providers were encouraged to stop treating themselves as "little entities" (Commissioner 3, CCG1, April 2014) in a competitive game looking after their own interests and to start acknowledging that lack of money in the local health system required a change of mentality (as well as more efficient processes). The way the case study sites embarked upon tackling such challenges was by talking with existing providers, gathering intelligence and data needed for service reviews, assessing the performance of services and areas that required change and finally looking for contractual levers to use to deliver the change. Going to the open market was seen as an option of last resort in respect of big service delivery transformations, and collaborative methods were preferred.

Although competition was not used to bring about large-scale service reconfigurations, commissioners in the case study sites did use competition for the market, using competitive tendering, in respect of smaller services. The services which were put out to tender were mostly primary care, community and diagnostic services. Individual services delivered in acute hospital settings were not often tendered, and no services in a whole hospital had been subject to competitive tendering.

Commissioners were asked to relate their experiences of tendering out a service, once they had decided on this route. Some commissioners stressed the importance of testing the market prior to issuing a formal invitation to tender. This was seen as necessary to ascertain provider interest in order to avoid the situation of having to go through a costly tendering process to end up with the same or a worse quality provider. Hosting provider engagement events was seen not only as a way to gauge provider interest, but also served as a general tool for mobilising existing providers to improve their performance. The use of adverts and market engagement events was a warning sign for incumbent providers that they ought to take commissioners seriously.

When assessing the bids, commissioners applied a number of criteria to assess the suitability of potential providers. In particular, they looked at whether providers were financially sustainable and capable of delivering the service.

Commissioners from CCG4 stated that they would have made more use of competitive tendering to procure services but felt constrained by the lack of resources to run such processes: "I would be more aggressive and probably more prone to tendering if I had more resource devoted to it and I would be moving resource from serious redesign or basic commissioning function into procuring and doing things in a more structured market interventionist way" (Commissioner 1, CCG4, November 2013). Most commissioners noted how time-consuming and expensive tendering was.

Providers were also asked about their experiences of participating in a tendering exercise. They reported that tendering was very resource intensive for them, and that it was made more difficult by the lack of experience of many commissioners. This affected the efficiency of the processes. Moreover, several providers were concerned that commissioners were relying on them to provide information required to write the tender specifications, rather than being able to do this themselves. Many providers noted that commissioners were still not able to specify the service at later stages of the process, and relied on each provider tendering to give details about what the service should comprise. This observation undermines the stated intention of the HSCA 2012 that GP commissioners would be setting the pace by specifying the services required for their local population.

Once the formal tendering process was underway, it was characterised by one provider as "chaotic" (Provider 1, NHS, acute, CCG1, April 2014) due to the short notice periods for submitting the paperwork. A common complaint was the large amount of resources that NHS providers had to dedicate to pursue competitive tenders. In fact, some providers could not afford to bid, due to their poor financial situations.

'I think the challenges are making sure that you have sufficient money to invest in bidding for things, because it takes a lot of time and effort, particularly from an Operational Team, a Clinical Team, but also the finance and information you support. And traditionally, you know, 'cause we don't have any money, we're poor, we don't have a budget set aside, so you're asking people to do it on top of their normal job.' (Provider 4, NHS, acute, CCG4, April 2014)

Often the information released by commissioners was not sufficient for a provider to make a cost–benefit assessment before deciding whether the tender would be viable.

As part of the research into how commissioners were using competition in the NHS, it was investigated whether CCGs had a strategy to develop the market for non-NHS independent providers. None of the sites had a deliberate strategy to enable greater involvement by for-profit providers in the provision of services. Instead, they appeared as contractors to the NHS on an ad hoc basis.

'We've used the independent sector to develop services that are substitutional for secondary care, or to outplace secondary care services. We've used them equally for some aspects of what's traditionally been community provision. So it's case by case. I don't think we have a — there isn't a kind of an overarching policy imperative to either grow or restrict the private sector. We use it where it's relevant.' (Commissioner 1, CCG2, November 2013)

Some commissioners were at pains to point out that they were careful to treat all providers equally, irrespective of whether they were NHS or not. One CCG (CCG4) was more enthusiastic about its entry into the NHS quasi-market than the others. On the other hand, all of the CCGs were actively engaged in supporting local third-sector organisations. Providers did not agree that they were all treated equally, and, in particular, some independent providers complained about being at a disadvantage. It appeared that, on the whole, small and medium-size independent providers did not experience the same level of communication and engagement from commissioners as larger independent providers or NHS trusts.

Apart from a specific local commissioning climate created by their main commissioning CCG (for example in CCG3, where the commissioners did not favour the use of competition), the different types of provider (acute, CHS and MHS) faced different constraining factors. Many of these constraints were determined at the national level — most importantly, different pricing mechanisms for different types of services. Furthermore, due to their different sizes, and the different types of services being delivered, the market horizon of some providers stretched beyond one particular CCG area to other CCGs and to markets created by different types of commissioning bodies, such as LAs. Thus, the position of a particular provider within the NHS was a product of a number of factors, such as the nature of the local market, the type of services it provided and whether it was able to reach other markets.

Providers in the study sites had first-hand experience of how the principles of competition and cooperation worked together in healthcare delivery practice. Providers had to comply with dual incentives to both cooperate and compete with other providers in the system and, importantly, to engage with commissioners in service planning. This led to circumstances in which providers sometimes collaborated with their competitors and competed with their collaborators. This applied to all types of provider, including independents.

Providers expressed concern about barriers preventing fair competition. One important issue was the different pricing mechanisms for acute and out-of-hospital care. An interviewee contrasted the position of MHS (which had block contracts, effectively a fixed budget) with that of the acute trusts, which could expand their provision due to being paid on a cost-per-case basis through PbR.

Whether competing or cooperating in respect of gaining (or trying not to lose) patients, all providers noted that they cooperated at the clinical level, to ensure that patients moved smoothly between organisations. Other reasons for collaborating included partnerships to deliver non-clinical services; participating in local service transformation programmes; and forming partnerships to compete for tenders.

In addition to understanding how providers both competed and cooperated with each other in the case study sites, it was important to understand providers' perceptions of their relationships with the commissioners. It was found that, in different circumstances, providers experienced both threats of competition and encouragement to collaborate with the commissioners and each other. They took the view that both of these techniques were being used by commissioners to influence their behaviour, and thus improve services. Providers of services out of hospital were more susceptible to threats of tendering than acute providers. CHS and MHS providers thought that the balance of power rested firmly with the commissioners. This is because CHS were more likely to be put out to tender and because block contract payments prevented expansion of services on providers' initiative.

However, all types of provider could see the advantages of being encouraged to collaborate, and of having good working relationships with their commissioners. These might even obviate the need for commissioners to put services out to tender.

Changes in behaviour following the publication of the FYFV

The FYFV (2014) emphasised the need for NHS organisations to cooperate with each other, and did not appear to favour the use of competition as a mechanism to improve services.

The follow-up interviews conducted in 2015 painted a mixed picture of commissioning practices in the four case study sites. On the one hand, all the case study sites were undertaking major local service transformation using collaborative working with providers (and had been doing so before the FYFV was published).

On the other hand, all four sites were using competitive tendering to procure some smaller, more peripheral services. This use of competition included CCG3, which reported the most collegial and collaborative commissioning culture in the initial interviews. By 2015 CCG3 had also been using a full procurement route for commissioning some of the services which experienced "poor quality, poor outcomes" issues (Commissioner 1, CCG3, July 2015) or in order to increase patient choice. The CCG3 commissioner had found the competitive approach useful as it injected new ideas into a "very conservative" local landscape (Commissioner 1, CCG3, July 2015).

Although noticing shifts in policy rhetoric towards cooperation following the FYFV, in their day-to-day practices commissioners were exercising their own judgement and making use of all tools available to them. In fact, taking account of CCG3, it can be seen that, over time, a wider range of commissioning mechanisms were being utilised.

Competition was being used alongside work on various projects to integrate services. However, the problem was how to integrate different work streams under one strategy.

> 'You've got to understand how many bids there are going on, and that's the confusing thing. We're a pioneer. [Acute trusts] are a vanguard for the care homes. I believe they've got a bid in as well with a group of other providers around something else, and there's so many things going off at the moment it's hard to keep a track.' (Commissioner 1, CCG1, August 2015)

In the interviews conducted during 2017 participants outlined some new commissioning practices which emerged as a result of widening disjuncture between the national legislation and policy. In addition to traditional competitive tendering used infrequently for relatively small community-based services, commissioners and providers reported the increasing use of 'hybrid' forms of competitive tendering. This referred to the open procurement processes which were conducted on the basis of existing competitive procurement guidance and infrastructure but which explicitly aimed at putting in place a collaborative arrangement between identified providers for provision of a particular type of service. This type of procurement utilised some elements of the competitive procurement process, such as open advertisements, but effectively required successful bidders to come together at some point in the process to propose a collaborative model of service delivery.

Such creative uses of the procurement framework by commissioners to "procure collaboration" (Commissioner 1, CCG2, June 2017) had an impact on provider behaviour. Interviewed providers noted that some commissioners preferred to receive joint bids from a number of provider organisations offering the right skill mix and, at the same time, have one organisation taking the lead to reduce fragmentation in the supply chain. Such commissioners' approach promoted collaboration between providers.

Unlike straightforward competitive procurement exercises, "procuring collaboration" was often associated with larger services and whole service lines. These procurements were often carried out jointly with other CCGs, making the whole process even more complex, with transaction costs potentially surpassing those of traditional competitive tendering.

Alongside the new 'hybrid' commissioning mechanisms, the CCGs continued to make use of a more traditional form of competitive tendering on an ad hoc and small-scale basis. Where full competitive procurement was used, it was usually because of the perceived availability of a number of potential providers and for fear of falling foul of the procurement rules. The high transaction costs associated with tendering continued to accompany traditional competitive tendering processes, with both commissioners and providers devoting substantial resources to preparing tenders and responding to the bids. Some commissioners reflected on the existing path dependency in the system, in that services that had been competitively tendered in the past were likely to require a repeat tendering following the expiry of the current contractual arrangement. Some commissioners and providers also noted difficulties with the mobilisation stage following traditional competitive procurements. For instance, this characterised a case where an independent provider won a tender at the expense of an incumbent NHS provider with which it had to cooperate on a care pathway.

There was also evidence of commissioners continuing to use procurement processes as a way of learning to specify and price a particular service. Interviewed providers found such practices frustrating and counterproductive, often resulting in iterative, protracted, start–stop types of procurement processes, whereby commissioners used the learning from the previous stage of procurement to inform their next steps.

The 2017 interviews indicated a notable change in the type of commissioning body in respect of competitive tendering in the four case study sites. The bulk of competitive tenders that providers responded to were instigated by the LA commissioners in charge of public health as opposed to CCG commissioners. Participants noted that, in contrast to CCG commissioners, LAs used competitive tendering almost as a "default option" (Provider 2, NHS, acute, CCG4, June 2017). Thus

LA commissioning became an important source of business for the interviewed providers. However, providers complained about the lack of market stewardship by LAs and ever-reducing financial envelopes. Providers also noted that fragmentation of commissioning between NHS and LA in services such as sexual health or children's services continued to pose problems.

CHS and MHS providers continued to be more affected by the competition for the market compared with the acute providers. Furthermore, some interviewed acute providers had begun to scale back internal resources dedicated to scanning for tendering opportunities and had become more selective about the type of tenders that they were prepared to respond to, developing niche specialisms. The acute providers perceived other acute providers more as collaborators than competitors and turned their focus to exploring new governance and clinical cooperation arrangements, including mergers and acquisitions, alliances and hospital chains. This marked a change from the findings from the earlier waves of fieldwork. The trend towards greater selectivity when bidding for contracts and exploring merger and collaboration arrangements was also visible in respect of some interviewed CHS and MHS providers. The selectivity was largely induced by the inadequate pricing of some of the contracts which the CHS and MHS providers were not prepared to (or could not afford to) provide at a loss. At the same time, CHS providers were still mindful of keeping track of opportunities to compete for services in order to retain their dominant position in their area. This meant that the CHS trusts simultaneously competed and collaborated with the same providers, even when going through mergers or preparing joint responses to bids.

> 'It's a really fine balance. So, yes, we do, I think in particular at STP level, we are then cooperating, you know, across patient pathways of mental health, whilst at the same time potentially competing against an organisation for a council commissioned service that's gone out to tender, so yes, we do both. So we'd be competing, yes, we'd be competing with an organisation at the same time as collaborating with them.' (Provider 2, NHS, CHS and/or MH, CCG1, June 2017)

By 2017, there was a growing acceptance amongst some providers of the overall responsibility of the local NHS for provision of vital services to the population, even if such services were unprofitable. According to some interviewed providers, joint responsibility and accountability for local health systems not only entailed commissioners eschewing competitive tendering which could undermine key local providers, but also put responsibility on the providers to continue offering services which were vital to the population, even if they might be unprofitable.

The latter dilemma related to the direct costs of cooperation in the context of tight financial resources, for instance the costs associated with taking over the deficits of struggling providers. Thus, although the ethos of the NHS as having cradle-to-grave responsibility for population health was posited by some participants as a factor differentiating the approach of NHS and independent providers, at the same time the NHS providers begun to feel the effects of the push towards collaboration by having to take on more financial risks.

> 'Whilst competition is a very overtly costly process, collaboration, in terms of some of the softer skills and, you know, one-to-one meetings and all those sorts of things, particularly if you're talking about collaborations across multiple organisations, not just one-to-one, actually, is very time intensive and because it's time intensive, then of course, it's – there's a cost attached to that 'cause it's just something that you're not doing then, elsewhere. So, for us, in particular, because we operate across a number of health systems, that's actually quite challenging.' (Provider 1, NHS, CHS and/or MH, CCG3, June 2017)

Independent providers were wary of the turn towards cooperative mechanisms in commissioning services as it would decrease their opportunities for market entry. Yet at the same time some independent providers had begun to explore working in partnership with NHS providers as another way of gaining market entry, for instance through STP structures. Private for-profit providers continued to be critical of how competition has been applied in the NHS, in particular with regard to a lack of a level playing field with NHS organisations in some aspects, and with regard to attitudes of and relationships with NHS commissioners and providers.

Conclusion

This research provided a unique insight into the local commissioning practices of NHS commissioners in England between 2013 and 2017, in respect of the use of competitive and collaborative commissioning levers. The research yielded rich, contextualised qualitative data on the understanding of the regulations and interpretation of policy signals by local commissioners as well as on commissioning practices and the rationale accompanying those practices.

Notwithstanding these advantages, the study has certain limitations. First, it should be noted that the study was not designed to assess the scale of the use of competitive and cooperative mechanisms in the NHS, or the actual effects of competition and cooperation on service efficiency, quality or patient outcomes. Second, the case study sites each represented a unique demographic and service configuration context, thus any trends uncovered here may not extend to the NHS as a whole. The unique setting of each case study site also made straightforward cross-case study comparisons problematic. Third, it should be noted that comparative data was not collected about the amount of resources available to be spent on procurement in each case study CCG. It was therefore impossible to speculate about whether there were differences which might have affected the CCGs' behaviour, in addition to other factors such as local market structure and attitudes of senior commissioning staff. Finally, persisting difficulties were encountered in appraising the number and value of services put out to competitive tendering, both at national and local levels. Gathering such intelligence required triangulation of many data sources, as there was no one place that held comprehensive information on the issue. It was found that such an aim was made even more complicated by the recent blurring of the distinction between the 'traditional' and 'hybrid' uses of competitive procurement process, which made it difficult to judge whether the process constituted competitive tendering or not.

Following the HSCA 2012 coming into force in April 2013, commissioners and providers found the provisions dealing with the procurement of clinical services confusing. The Act stipulated both competition and cooperation among providers. Participants also found that regulators such as Monitor were unhelpful in clarifying the ambiguity around application of the rules in particular cases.

Overall, collaboration was a preferred and default mode of operation for both commissioners and providers. Yet at the same time, some NHS commissioners, although critical of some aspects of competition, wanted to retain competitive mechanisms in the array of commissioning levers available to them.

Faced with ambiguity of legal and regulatory landscape, local commissioners as policy implementers exercised a lot of discretion in terms of which commissioning mechanism to use in particular circumstances. Arguably, it might have been the intention of policy makers to leave the justification of the method of commissioning to the local level. Yet there were also some limits to such discretion. Commissioners had to follow transparent procurement processes, be aware of any potential legal challenges, and be mindful of their position in the NHS managerial hierarchy. Therefore commissioners remained highly attuned to national policy messages and local providers' situations when deciding whether to put a particular service out to tender.

Overall, it was found that competitive mechanisms coexisted with cooperative mechanisms of commissioning services in all four case study sites, albeit the latter prevailed. Competitive tendering was also used as a threat to incentivise behaviour change amongst existing providers. Furthermore a twofold disjuncture was observed between the rules and practices of commissioning. At the outset of the fieldwork the rules were interpreted as stipulating competition whilst commissioners continued to work in their preferred collaborative commissioning mode and resisted 'enforced' competition where possible. Towards the end of the fieldwork the essence of the disjuncture changed in that commissioners were more open towards and encouraged to practice collaborative commissioning but felt unsupported by the legislation.

The findings of this research point to a clear policy challenge. Commissioners still wanted to be able to use competitive mechanisms of commissioning clinical services in some circumstances. Some local commissioners were still concerned that procurement rules stipulating competition ought to be taken into account. These attitudes appeared to conflict with the statements by NHSE and DH which were anti-competition in tone, including those by Simon Stevens (Dunhill, 2016; Thomas and West, 2017) and Jeremy Hunt (Lintern, 2017). Interviewed commissioners pointed out that using rhetoric to influence practice might only go so far in overcoming the implementation challenges, especially with regard to such complex issues as ACOs. Thus the study uncovered a pressing need for better alignment between the legal framework and the policy messages. It may be politically unpalatable, but the regulatory framework of the HSCA 2012 needs revisiting to ensure that commissioners have a clear choice about whether to use competitive mechanisms or not.

In addition, local commissioners should be allowed to make their own decisions about which modes of commissioning are most appropriate in their particular circumstances, and in respect of particular services. Setting up nationally imposed rules about what mechanisms must be used is unhelpful (and probably will not be adhered to). At the same time, it is important to clarify the rules of the game for local actors, in order for them to feel fully supported in the commissioning choices that they make.

7

Healthcare contracts and the allocation of financial risk

Pauline Allen, Marie Sanderson, Christina Petsoulas and Ben Ritchie

Introduction

Contracts, which were introduced into the English NHS in the early 1990s, are the crux of the internal market. As in all markets, the negotiation and implementation of contracts for healthcare allow purchasers and providers to exchange information, and provide a framework for the allocation of financial risk. Financial risk, here defined as uncertainty of outcome, is allocated between purchasers and providers to reconcile their potentially conflicting objectives. Effective risk allocation occurs when risk is allocated to those who can control it, thereby incentivising those with responsibility for the risk to act to mitigate it. The contractual financial levers of pricing and payment structures play a key role in the allocation of financial risk between buyers and sellers. In the NHS, pricing and payment structures can allocate financial risk between those commissioning and providing services in order to incentivise demand management, improve efficiency, and, through the use of risk-sharing arrangements, encourage providers to work collectively.

This chapter examines two studies of NHS contracting conducted by PRUComm which examine how pricing and payment structures in NHS contracts allocate financial risk. As outlined in Chapter 1, institutional economics and socio-legal concepts underlie the study's approach to understanding the use of contracts in the NHS quasi-market. Contracting for health is challenging because of the complexity of health services and concomitant high levels of asymmetric information and uncertainty between providers of care and its purchasers (Arrow, 1963). Opportunism may occur as a result of this 'information impactedness' (Williamson, 1975), and one party may take advantage of the other's information deficit. Higher levels of asymmetric information will result in higher costs of negotiating and writing contracts, as well as monitoring, enforcing and renegotiating them. The purchaser can use the mechanisms of the contract, such as pricing and payment structures, to encourage the provider to deliver the outcomes desired by the purchaser, and to try to overcome the problems caused by imperfect information. Relational norms of contracts allow adjustments to be made to the initially agreed terms during the course of the contractual relationship to deal with unforeseen contingencies (Vincent-Jones, 2006).

The examination of the negotiation, specification and monitoring of contracts in practice is important because it is misleading simply to analyse the formal provisions of the contract alone, as actual practice often does not comply with contractual rules (Macneil, 1981). Research has shown that the operation of contracts in the NHS tends to entail flexibility, and there may well be changes in the terms of the contractual relationship which are at odds with the written document signed by the parties (as was discussed in more detail in Chapter 1). This phenomenon indicates that research is required to investigate how the NHS contractual mechanisms, including financial levers to allocate risk, are working in practice. For example, research on NHS contractual governance which investigated the first few years of the standard contract indicated that actual allocation of financial risk deviated in practice from that set out in the contractual documents, and thus national pricing rules were not always followed (Petsoulas et al, 2011).

The two studies reported here present two differing ways in which NHS contracting deals with the allocation of risk. The first study, which is based an examination of the NHS standard contract from 2011 to 2015, investigates how commissioners negotiated, specified, monitored and managed contractual mechanisms in the NHS standard contract to allocate financial risk in their local health economies and improve services. The second, more recent, study (2016–18) concerns the adoption of new forms of contractual arrangements in the NHS, such as alliance agreements, which aim to incentivise providers of health and/or care services to work together to achieve a common aspiration through the sharing of financial risk. Whilst these studies present different perspectives on the allocation of risk in NHS contracts, they are illustrative of the enduring challenges facing both commissioners and providers in allocating financial risk in a way which does not impede integration and innovation.

Pricing and payment structures in the English NHS

As described in Chapter 2, the pricing and payment structures which can be used in relation to the provision of services in the English NHS are set by the hierarchy. There is, importantly, no price competition. Pricing in the English NHS is mainly (although not entirely) stipulated in the terms of the NHS standard contract. However, limited flexibilities in the pricing and payment structures are available to commissioners.

The three main types of payment mechanisms for the provision of English NHS services (block contracts, cost and volume contracts and cost per case) allocate financial risk in differing ways. Block contracts, for example, allocate the risk of overperformance to service providers, while the use of cost-per-case mechanisms allocate the risk of overperformance to the purchaser (and underperformance to the provider). In some instances the nature of the services being contracted for necessitates a specific type of payment mechanism, for example currently there is no tariff available for CHS and MHS, and commissioners should negotiate local payments in the form of a block contract. Additionally, NHS standard contracts may specify local variations to payment, such as quality payments and financial penalties that provide incentives to achieve specific targets. Local 'modifications' are also allowed in the case of unavoidable higher local costs. The differences between these payment mechanisms furnish commissioners with a way to encourage desired provider behaviour, for instance around demand management.

The FYFV (NHS England, 2014a) has led to policy developments which entail separate organisations working closely together to improve the integration of local services, such as ICSs, STPs, and the exploration of new models of care through the Vanguard programme. A fundamental element underlying such integration policies is the development of new contractual models which can underpin and facilitate closer working between organisations, and which allow greater flexibility in the allocation of resources in local health economies. New contractual models, such as alliance contracting and lead provider contracting, attempt to share (some or all) financial risk between a group of providers. These new contractual models give organisations the opportunity to explore new payment systems and risk-sharing arrangements on a limited basis, through the use of payment mechanisms such as multilateral gain/loss sharing, capitated payments and outcome-based payments, which seek to achieve unity of purpose by sharing financial risk amongst providers.

Pricing and the allocation of financial risk

The first study described in this chapter is a unique examination of the changes in the NHS national pricing rules and the actual allocation of financial risk on the ground during the four financial years 2011–12 to 2014–15. This period is particularly interesting as the regulatory framework for the NHS was altered by the coming into force of the HSCA 2012 in April 2013, which created an economic regulator (Monitor) and extended competition law (and thus the jurisdiction of the national competition authorities) to apply to the planning and provision of NHS services (Sanderson et al, 2017). Prior to the introduction of the HSCA, prices had been subject to flexibility in practice (Monitor, 2013a). It has been argued that the introduction of the new regime under the HSCA would have the effect of juridifying decision making, thus removing the internal flexibility previously enjoyed by the NHS (Davies, 2013). The rationale for this was that, in order to produce a level playing field between all types of provider (including independent ones), it was necessary for pricing rules to be transparent and applied equally to all providers.

The study investigated how commissioners negotiated, specified, monitored and managed contractual mechanisms to improve services and allocate financial risk in their local health economies, looking at both acute services and community health care. Both the changing contractual provisions and the behaviour of contracting parties at local level were examined. The key questions this research addressed was to establish the range of formal provisions, including positive and negative financial levers in respect of quality of care in contracts across the English NHS; how contractual financial levers were negotiated, specified, monitored and enforced in practice; how prices were set, and what payments were actually made to providers.

The project consisted of three aspects. Firstly, there was a detailed analysis of each year's standard NHS national contract from 2011–12 to 2014–15. Secondly, there were two national telephone surveys of commissioners in 2012 and 2014 to find out what pricing mechanisms were being used in formal written contracts, and how they were implemented (or not). Thirdly, a series of three in-depth case studies of three local health economies were conducted, looking at the contractual relationships between commissioning organisations and their providers of acute, MH and community healthcare. These consisted of interviews with 27 contracting personnel in commissioners and providers, observations of 21 contracting meetings and analysis of local documents. This triangulated approach permitted a broader and more reliable picture of the findings: the surveys helped put the case studies within the overall national context, whereas the case studies enabled the research questions to be examined in greater depth.

The study found a marked difference between the rules promulgated at national level and the allocation of financial risk by local actors. These findings are to be expected, given the well-known difficulties in contracting for healthcare, and the continuing influence of hierarchical factors (in particular the cash-limited budget) on the NHS quasi-market.

Provisions of the national standard contracts

The relevant provisions of the national standard contracts remained relatively stable during the research period until 2014–15, when greater local financial flexibility was permitted. For acute services, the contract provided for the use of both national tariff (formerly PbR) prices and the negotiation of local prices in respect of care which was not covered by it.

Although the principle behind the use of PbR was that providers should be paid for every episode of care delivered, the 2011–12 national contract included limits on activity which would be reimbursed. Commissioners could refuse to pay for more activity than had been forecast. After 2012, this contractual provision was deleted because the then economic regulator, the CCP, ruled that commissioners could not place a cap on activity, as it restricted patient choice. Nevertheless, each year's contract provided that emergency admissions exceeding a local baseline figure from 2008 to 2009 would only be reimbursed at 30 per cent of tariff.

The 2014–15 contract, for the first time, contained provisions specifically designed to allow the parties greater flexibility in pricing. 'Local variations' were designed to allow adjustments to prices or currencies to facilitate significant service redesign or reconfiguration. 'Local modifications' were allowed in the case of unavoidable higher local costs. Moreover, for 2014–15 the contract allowed the parties to vary the baseline figure over which emergency activity would be reimbursed at 30 per cent. The standard contract did not contain pricing rules for MH and community services – these were negotiated locally in the form of block contracts.

Negotiation, monitoring and enforcement of contracts

The data collected in the surveys and the case studies were similar, allowing them to be reported together, and conclusions to be drawn that are likely to apply across the English NHS. In respect of contracts between CCGs and NHS acute trusts, the allocation of financial risk outside the framework of the various formal pricing mechanisms was striking. Most of the contractual relationships between NHS acute providers and commissioners were characterised by the use of general annual financial settlements outside the terms of the contract. Whatever detailed financial provisions had been agreed and implemented during the course of the year, a final overall agreement was made at year-end which did not adhere strictly to the contractual provisions. It was not always possible for commissioners to pay the full contractually designated amount for activity undertaken, as their budgets were insufficient. This appeared to be increasing over time, with more commissioners reporting not being able to afford to pay the full amount for the level of activity provided by the time of the second survey in mid-2014. Year-end deals were seen as pragmatic and inevitable in the context of the NHS:

> 'Well, this is, you see, this is where PbR shows its – how can I say? – its limitations. At the end of the day, health economies need to be in balance ... it's in nobody's interests to bankrupt any of the parties associated with the relevant health economy, and that's almost a diktat in terms of public policy, OK?' (Case Study B, Commissioning Consultant, Commissioning Support Unit)

But there was variation between the commissioners that responded. Several confirmed that they simply followed the contract and paid for all activity undertaken, even if it was more than they expected. These were areas where there was sufficient money available to commissioners for them to afford to do so. The new provisions in the 2014–15 contract allowing for variation in allocation of financial risk were used by some CCGs, although by no means the majority. This was because other commissioners continued to make informal arrangements to allocate risk at the end of the financial year, and did not see any point in formalising these by notifying national regulators. Three commissioners had used the new provisions allowing for flexibility in national tariff prices ('local variations'). One had submitted variations in relation to six tariff areas to Monitor. The provider was a tertiary hospital and the new approach was needed due to the fact that NHSE had taken over commissioning of some of the services. Variations to national tariffs were needed to keep within the CCG budget. Another commissioner had agreed a lower local tariff with its provider if a patient was admitted for less than two hours, which was sent to NHSE and Monitor for agreement.

A few parties ignored the national instructions on pricing and agreed a block contract for all acute services at the beginning of the financial year in 2012 and 2014. This was because they could foresee that the local health economy could not bear the cost of PbR, with unlimited financial exposure for the commissioners. Not all of these agreements were reported to Monitor. By 2014, some commissioners had reported these to NHSE as 'local modifications'. One commissioner explained that they might be forming an integrated care organisation, and this, in addition to the financial risks to the acute provider posed by transferring money to the local Better Care Fund (that is, out of the acute sector), required different payment provisions.

There was a conflict between different policy objectives: financial solvency for each NHS provider trust on the one hand; and reconfiguring services so that more care is provided outside hospital on the other. One CCG director of finance pointed out:

> 'We did look, this year, at trying to move the acute trust contract away from PbR to more caps and collars [that is, block] contract base, but, again, the trust development agency [that is, national regulatory agency] were not supportive with that approach. Because the acute trust is financially challenged, they didn't want them to do that. But the only way we're going to be able to redesign services and reduce the secondary care footprint is to try and take some of the discussion away from finance and prices to an agreement where we have a set level of income for a set level of activity and we collectively work together to step it down because the PbR system and the contracting is slightly perverse in that why would the acute trust want to step down activity when it gets paid for what it delivers?' (Case Study A, Director of Finance, CCG)

Despite the increased flexibility in the 2014–15 contract, most of the commissioners were still using the 2008–09 baseline for setting the point at which the 30 per cent marginal rate for emergency admissions applied. Several had moved to later figures. One commissioner had done so because there had been major changes in the configuration of acute services since 2008–09. Other commissioners had moved to later baselines, such as 2011–12, in one case after having been forced to do so following arbitration. In some places, commissioners felt obliged to pay so-called 'non-recurring' additional amounts to their NHS acute providers in order to help the hospitals balance their books at the end of the year. This was related to the need in some areas to facilitate the reconfiguration of local services, which might require transitional payments to support changes in service delivery in the short term. This could only occur in areas where commissioners had sufficient additional funds available.

It was investigated how prices for non-tariff activity were agreed. In 2012 in most areas, prices paid the previous year were reduced by the current NHS-wide efficiency target. By 2014, a wider range of techniques was in use. In a few areas, there were attempts to benchmark local prices with those in other areas. Very rarely there were attempts to undertake more accurate costing exercises in respect of some of these services. These were undertaken in areas where there was particular concern that current prices were inaccurate. In addition, by 2014–15, increasing numbers of commissioners were insisting on agreeing a fixed sum in respect of these non-PbR services – effectively another block contract. This was related to the poor financial situation in those areas, where money had to be saved in order to try to stay within commissioning budgets. In contrast to the behaviour with NHS providers, all commissioners reported being able to pay independent providers of acute services in accordance with the PbR rules. This may have been due to the fact that there were insignificant volumes of such activity, so the financial viability of the local health economy was not threatened. Block contracts were used in respect of CHS and MH services, in accordance with national contracting rules.

Volumes of activity were monitored throughout the year and any over- or underperformance informed the setting of the next year's block amount. Although the block contract limited financial risk for commissioners, it also impeded moving the activity from one type of provider (for example acute trust) to another (for example community healthcare setting), which was a national policy priority. In order to make such moves easier, the participants suggested that national tariffs were needed in respect of CHS, so that money would follow the patient:

> 'There's something about as we move forward, we recognise that we've got to transform services. So essentially, less direct acute provision and more alternative provision, either a primary care, community care or social care setting. Now, in order for that to happen, it's simpler that the money follows the patient. So from that perspective, I think, going forward, a tariff type contract works better, because the money's more easily moved.' (Case Study C, Director of Finance, CCG)

Context for contracting

The context in which the contractual relationships that were studied took place was very important. First, the case studies demonstrated that personal relationships between staff were a vital element in facilitating effective contractual relationships. The degree of flexibility required could only be achieved where these worked well. Second, the increasing financial stringency affecting the whole NHS during the course of the study had an effect on the way in which the contracts could be used at local level. As less money was available, it became increasingly difficult for commissioners to adhere to the national tariff rules. Third, in the later years of the study, national and local policies entailed major service reconfigurations at local level, mainly aimed at shifting resources from acute care to social care and CHS. The contractual pricing rules impeded this.

New models of NHS contract: the allocation of risk across providers

The study of pricing reported on pages 106–111 illustrates how financial risk in the period in question was handled differently in practice from formal contractual provisions. Despite new pricing flexibilities in the NHS standard contract, increasing numbers of commissioners and NHS acute providers were agreeing to abandon the national tariff and settle on a block contract (that is, a fixed budget) in order to limit the financial risk to the commissioners. By 2014–15, increasing numbers of local contracts contained block contract provisions for services not covered by the national tariff, rather than any form of pricing for activity.

One issue raised by the study related to the difficulties of achieving service improvement and innovation in a contractual environment which did not support the movement of activity between providers. The second study in this chapter explores new models of NHS contracting which attempt to allocate financial risk amongst providers in order to address such issues.

New models of contracting in the NHS

Following the publication of the FYFV (NHS England, 2014a) contractual models to encourage integration have been developed. These have the status of voluntary contractual options to be selected locally depending on which contractual solution is deemed likely to work best given local circumstances. Risk sharing has previously been permissible on a binary basis (between commissioner and provider) within the terms of the NHS standard contract (Allen et al, 2014b) for use during a period of significant service reconfiguration. New contractual models such as alliance contracting and lead provider contracting attempt to share financial risk between a group of providers. An NHS Alliance agreement brings providers together around a common aspiration for joint working across the system. The agreement does not replace or in any way override existing Service Contracts, such as the NHS standard contract. The Alliance agreement sets out a number of shared objectives and principles, and a set of shared governance rules allowing providers to come together to take decisions (NHS England, 2017d). A NHS lead provider arrangement is one in which a single provider entity takes full contractual responsibility, through a Service Contract, for the delivery of a range of integrated services for a specific population (NHS England, 2015a).

Like many of the initiatives which are currently exploring integration across providers, such new contractual models give commissioners and providers the opportunity to explore new payment systems and risk-sharing arrangements on a limited basis which seek to encourage rather than inhibit integration. This may be achieved through the use of payment mechanisms such as multilateral gain/loss sharing, capitated payments and outcome-based payments. All these mechanisms seek to achieve unity of purpose by sharing financial risk amongst providers.

Multilateral gain/loss share arrangements can be deployed to share financial risk between organisations (Monitor, 2015c). Multilateral gain/loss share arrangements aim to realign the financial incentives of individual organisations to improve the delivery of outcomes for the whole system. They can also protect providers from a sudden loss in revenue or from an unpaid increase in activity. This is achieved by allowing (multiple) commissioners and providers to distribute any savings and losses from system change among themselves, thereby mitigating financial risk and incentivising the achievement of system rather than organisational goals.

Capitation is a means of paying a provider or group of providers to cover the majority (or all) of the care provided to a target population across different care settings (Monitor, 2014a). If the specified care is provided to the target population for less than the capitated payment, the financial gain generated is retained. This approach is thought to incentivise providers to deliver proactive care to patients, identify risks earlier and arrange the most effective care for patients. The risk in this approach lies with the providers that have to manage their activity within a fixed cost, and the rationale is that it realigns the financial risk with the parties that deliver care.

Risk/reward shared incentive structures divide financial rewards and penalties according to a fixed pre-agreed ratio between providers to reflect performance against targets. Outcome-based payments link a share of the payment to the achievement of defined outcomes (in place of payment for processes such as numbers of episodes of care delivered). Outcome-based payment can be linked to many other payment mechanisms, and can be used to incentivise service provision across a number of providers. Where the outcome payments relate to a contractual arrangement linking providers together, this arrangement incentivises providers to work together to achieve system outcomes. Outcome-based payments may have varying degrees of relative importance within the contract dependent on the proportion of the overall payment which is dedicated to performance in relation to outcomes.

Background

Three in-depth case studies were conducted to investigate how such new models of contracting were being implemented in the NHS. The research explored why commissioners chose to adopt new models of contracting, the characteristics of these new contractual documents, including payment structures; and how the new contractual models contributed to the reconfiguration of services in local health economies. The study was interested in how the contracts addressed issues associated with financial risk generally, including relevant payment structures. The descriptions of payment structures in the contractual documentation were reviewed, and interviewees were also asked to describe how payment structures operated in practice.

The fieldwork took place in two phases. The first round of interviews across three case studies took place between October 2016 and June 2017, and the second round took place between April 2018 and July 2018. Two of the case studies (A and B) concerned the development and use of Alliance agreements. The third case study (C) was based on the long-term aim of the agreement of a lead provider contractual arrangement with a population-based/capitated payment mechanism with outcome payments. In the first phase of the research representatives of all contractual (or proposed contractual) partners in the three case studies were interviewed – a total of 20 people (in 17 interviews). In the second phase of the research eight people were interviewed (in seven interviews). The purpose of the second round of data collection was to gauge how the new contractual models were developing over time. The fieldwork consisted of three main activities: the documents which supported the new contractual arrangements were analysed; the relevant senior managers of the organisations which were party to the contracts were interviewed; meetings of the contracting parties at which they specified and monitored performance in relation to the new contractual models were observed.

The contractual arrangements in two of the case studies (A and C) were under negotiation at the start of the research, whilst the other contractual model (Case Study B Alliance agreement) had been in operation for nearly two years. The contractual arrangements varied greatly in scope and value (see Table 7.1).

The proposed Alliance agreement in Case Study A was the most ambitious venture, between the commissioners and providers of social care and NHS-funded healthcare services to people aged 65 and over living in the LA area, and related to service contracts together worth approximately £200 million in the first year. It was hoped the Alliance would facilitate service redesign leading to 10–15 per cent savings in relation to spend on over 65s across the lifetime of the contract. The Alliance agreement in Case Study B related to the delivery of services and support for people with severe MH problems, and focused on the use of rehabilitation inpatient beds or residential placements in the LA area. It was the progression of informal partnership working between the commissioner and provider members in relation to similar services. The contractual arrangement was anticipated to achieve 25 per cent savings targets on an approximately £12 million budget. Case Study C was based on the long-term aim of the agreement of a lead provider contractual arrangement with a population-based/capitated payment mechanism with outcome payments for the provision of adult out-of-hospital care (CHS) and social care services in a LA area. When the research commenced it had not been possible to reach agreement between local providers about this proposed model, so numerous contracts and schedules were put in place to underpin the future development of the contractual arrangement. The first stage of this arrangement related to a NHS standard contract, worth approximately £20 million in the first year, for community adult healthcare services and local commissioned (GP) services between the community NHS Trust and the CCG. A Joint Venture agreement and a standard NHS subcontract existed between the community NHS Trust and the General Practice Alliance for the development and delivery

Table 7.1: Contractual arrangements by case study (as at the start of the research period)

Case Study	Model	Services	Participants	Value – Yr 1	Payment structures
A	Alliance agreement	Health and social care services to the over 65s	- CCG - LA - NHS Trust 1 - NHS Trust 2 - GP collaborative - Third-sector organisation	£200 million	Current: Mixture of PbR and block Intended: Capitation (mechanism to be agreed during Year 1) with proportion of payment on basis of outcomes. Multilateral risk share.
B	Alliance agreement	MH (provision of rehabilitation inpatient beds or residential placements)	- CCG - LA - NHS Trust - Third-sector organisation 1 - Third-sector organisation 2	£12 million	Monthly payments based on forecast activity with proportion of payment on basis of outcomes. Multilateral risk share.
C	Joint venture agreement/MoU for further contractual model	Adult out of hospital care and social care services	- Joint venture agreement - Community trust - GP federation - With 'MoU partners' - Acute NHS FT - Acute NHS FT - LA - CCG	£20 million	Current: Block payment to community trust Intended: Intend to move to population based/capitated payment mechanism and with proportion of payment on basis of outcomes.

of community adult healthcare services and local commissioned (GP) services. A wider group of parties signed a Memorandum of Understanding (MoU) committing to the development of the desired larger contractual arrangement.

Commissioners' aims in adopting these contractual models were to develop collective responsibility between providers for performance by transferring the risk to those who had the financial and service delivery levers to manage it. It was hoped that such agreements encompassing multiple providers would achieve transformational outcomes not encouraged through the sole use of bilateral contracts and payment mechanisms in relation to service redesign and financial savings. The study found that the negotiation of the allocation of financial risk through the new contractual models was a lengthy and complex process, and there was a tendency to defer decisions relating to the allocation of risk beyond the commencement of the contract. However the study also found that such new models of contracting are particularly valuable in terms of their capacity to establish trusting relationships and shared vision between providers.

Provisions of the contracts

The Alliance agreements in Case Studies A and B were based on the NHS Template Alliance agreement (NHS England, 2016b). The Alliance agreements, describing how organisations would work together, were 'wrapped around' bilateral NHS standard contracts for the services subject to the Alliance agreement. The division was described in both Alliance agreements as one in which the Alliance agreement describes how parties will work together in a collaborative and integrated way, and the NHS standard contracts describe how services will be provided. The case study Alliance agreements centred on the general principle that risks should be shared across alliance members and that no alliance member should derive unreasonable advantage or suffer unreasonable disadvantage. The Alliance agreements outlined the commitment of partners to work together, to take responsibility for making unanimous decisions on a best for services basis, to take collective ownership of risk and reward and to adopt 'an uncompromising commitment to trust, honesty, collaboration, innovation and mutual support' (Clause 7.1, Template Alliance agreement).

The contractual arrangements in Case Study C contained fewer general principles which directly addressed risk sharing. It was intended that the first year of the Joint Venture should be used to develop a wider contractual arrangement between the Joint Venture partners, two acute NHS Trusts and the LA which would include a capitated payment mechanism based on a fixed payment, an outcome-based incentive payment and a contingency.

Case Study B was the only arrangement in which the allocation of financial risk was specified in detail in the written contractual documents. In Case Studies A and C the sharing of financial risk among multiple partners through mechanisms such as capitated payments, payment on the basis of outcomes and multilateral gain/loss sharing was deferred beyond the commencement of the contractual arrangements. In Case Study B the Alliance agreement included a gain/pain share agreement consisting of a small number of financially incentivised outcome-based measures. These were in operation for Year Two onwards of the contract. The amount available for gain/pain share was worth just in excess of a modest 1 per cent (£140,000) of the £12 million contract value. The ratio of payment for both the gain and pain share related to each provider's proportion of the contract value (approximately 40 per cent each for the LA and the NHS FT, and 10 per cent each for both third-sector providers).

Additionally, the contract documentation addressed how the wider financial risks of the Alliance would be managed between the commissioners and providers, and between the groups of providers. This concerned firstly how any gains or losses relating to performance against the financial envelope would be managed and, secondly, how loss of revenue to particular providers as a result of service reconfiguration would be managed. The risk associated with overspending against the financial envelope sat with the Alliance providers, who had responsibility to resolve overspends and unanticipated demand without assistance from the commissioner, unless additional demand exceeded the activity and financial plan by 10 per cent or more. The agreement did not specify how this 'loss pool' should be shared proportionately between providers, and therefore it appeared that this should be agreed between Alliance partners when the situation arises. In relation to the sharing of underspends against the financial envelope, in Year One any cost reductions would be returned to the commissioners, and in subsequent years cost reductions would be firstly ploughed into service development, with any further remaining money split, with 50 per cent returned to the commissioners and 50 per cent made available to the providers.

The Alliance agreement explicitly recognised that the risks associated with shifting activity in the Case Study B service model rested with the MH NHS FT, which would experience a decrease in activity should the Alliance be successful. However, the written agreement did not address specifically how this risk should be shared apart from in the spirit of the general principle that risks should be shared across alliance members and that no alliance member should derive unreasonable advantage or suffer unreasonable disadvantage as a result of the work of the Alliance.

The allocation of financial risk in practice

In practice in the case studies the transfer and sharing of financial risk achieved through these new contractual models was limited.

In Case Studies A and C the contractual partners were unable to agree the means by which risks would be shared amongst them. When Case Study A was revisited at the end of the first year of the contract, it was reported that the Alliance partners had not agreed any new payment structures, and had not reached an agreement about the sharing of financial risk between providers. Similarly, in relation to Case Study C, outcome-based payments had not been put in place for the service contract to which the Joint Venture agreement related, and plans had not been progressed to establish a larger-scale contractual model with a wider group of providers based on outcome payments and a capitated population-based payment mechanism. Indeed, in both case studies whilst the contractual arrangements were still in place their remit had been substantially remodelled, and they were no longer seen as vehicles which would facilitate the allocation of financial risk amongst providers. In Case Study A, the Alliance had been subsumed into the wider work programme of the STP as a vehicle for the delivery of business cases. In Case Study C the contractual model was no longer supported by the CCG, which felt it was not sufficiently transformative in its aims, and not aligned to national policy concerning the integration of health and social care.

In Case Study B, however, it was possible to compare the allocation of financial risk in practice with the arrangements to share financial risk which had been agreed in the written contract.

The financial risk posed to commissioners and providers by the outcome-based payments was insignificant. The payments related to the achievement of outcomes accounted for only a small percentage of the financial envelope. This was described as a deliberate approach by both commissioners and providers: the incentive was kept small because of the limited contractual length (three years), because of the need to make savings within the financial envelope of the Alliance, and because the Alliance wished to trial the use of outcome-based payments. As this element was so small it was noted by interviewees that it was not a strong driver for performance

The allocation of financial risk in relation to over/underspends and activity changes due to service redesign was a more significant issue in practice, and there was evidence that the Alliance providers had successfully shared financial risk during the operation of the contract. As expected, due to the implementation of a new service model by the Alliance, the MH NHS FT had lost income as activity (and payment) shifted from inpatient beds to care delivered in community settings. In line with the general principle of the Alliance agreement that risks should be shared across alliance members and that no alliance member should derive unreasonable advantage or suffer unreasonable disadvantage as a result of the work of the Alliance, the alliance provider organisations netted off individual over/underspends at the end of the first year of the contract. In actuality these risks were split between the MH NHS FT and the LA, as the smaller contractual partners (the third-sector organisations) were considered exempt from the risk share arrangements.

Agreement of the allocation of financial risk

A number of factors appeared to influence the agreements which were reached in the case studies about the allocation of financial risks.

Firstly, tension regarding the 'shared ownership' of financial risk remained a significant stumbling block for provider organisations, in a wider institutional context in which individual NHS organisations were still individually regulated and held accountable for an individual 'financial control total' representing the minimum level of financial performance which their boards, governing bodies and chief executives must deliver each financial year. In light of the savings built into the financial models for each of the contractual arrangements, NHS organisations were aware that one or more of the contractual partners would suffer financially in order for the proposed service reconfigurations to work, whilst still being held accountable for their organisation's individual financial recovery plan. Whilst NHSI had recently introduced the concept of 'system-wide' financial control totals (which did not appear to be in place in the case studies), individual organisations were still to be held accountable for delivering both their individual control totals and also overall system control, unless special permission was granted (NHS England and NHS Improvement, 2016).

Concerns regarding individual organisational accountability were compounded by perceived uncertainty about the scope of the contractual arrangements. There were doubts about the accuracy and robustness of statutory sector financial and activity information systems, which consequently affected the robustness of financial models. There were associated concerns about whether financial models had been adequately stress tested (a risk management technique in which the potential impact of unlikely, although plausible, events or movements in a set of financial variables is tested). Interviewees also referred to a lack of clarity about the definitions of the services, patients and conditions to be included in the contractual arrangements. Such uncertainties were an issue across all three case study sites and all types of providers. Larger partners were concerned about the basis for the scale of the savings required of them, and it was feared that smaller partners did not have sufficient resources to compensate for inaccuracies in the model. One response to such uncertainties was withdrawal from the proposed contractual arrangement. Indeed in Case Study C, both the LA and the two acute trusts withdrew from the proposed contractual arrangement amid concerns that, firstly, the financial risk had not been adequately quantified and, secondly, that they would be obliged to bear too much risk.

Where agreement had been reached regarding the sharing of financial risk, and where financial risk had been shared in practice, there had been a reliance on relational norms of contracting. In Case Study B trusting and historical relationships between the Alliance partners were cited as crucial factors enabling the resolution of such issues within the life of the contract:

> 'We'd known each other for some time though, as people and organisations, because we'd done all the work with the [local collaborative initiative] and the [local group]. I think it would be different if we'd come cold to it. I think that's one of the problems that other Alliances may find if they're trying to pull together people who haven't worked together before.' (Mental Health Trust, Case Study B)

In the light of the difficulty of agreeing the written contractual arrangements for the allocation of financial risk, as evidenced by the problems related to the agreement of financial modelling, entering into such arrangements where risks were to be shared dynamically across providers during the life of the contract required an initial leap of faith based on trust in contractual partners. It is common practice in such models, particularly the Alliance model, for the governance structures to facilitate the formation and strengthening of close and trusting relationships between contractual partners (Langfield-Smith, 2008).

A clear strength of these models, particularly the Alliance model, was that they enabled the development of trusting and productive inter-organisational relationships between the parties. It was found that, despite the lack of agreement regarding the transfer of risk in Case Studies A and C, service providers had moved forward with service reconfiguration to a degree without changing pre-existing payment mechanisms, in the light of the more general commitments they had made to each other.

Discussion

The two studies described in this chapter examine ways in which contracting in the English NHS addresses the allocation of financial risk. The studies concern differing contractual arrangements and types of financial risk. The first study concerns the allocation of financial risk between a commissioner and provider within the terms of the NHS standard contract, and describes a dissonance between the rules promulgated at national level, and the local agreements which were put in place to manage risk. The second study explores new models of NHS contracting which are used to allocate financial risk to groups of providers, and describes the difficulty of agreeing the terms of such arrangements, and the flexibilities which are required during the life of the contract in practice.

Although they describe two different approaches to the allocation of financial risk, both studies indicate that the allocation of financial risk is dealt with outside the formal structures of the contract. Indeed, the extent to which the evidence about contracting for healthcare has been constant over the past two and a half decades is striking. It remains the case that formal contracts are not able to deal with all eventualities (as found earlier by, for example, Flynn et al, 1996; McHale et al, 1997; Allen, 2002b; Petsoulas et al, 2011), and that, in particular, allocation of financial risk is often dealt with outside the formal structures of the written document.

The introduction of new contractual models such as Alliance agreements and associated payment mechanisms such as multilateral gain/loss sharing constitutes a response to some of the problems encountered in relation to the allocation of financial risk, through the NHS standard contract described in the first study, and the creation of a contractual environment which facilitates service redesign and innovation by supporting the movement of activity between providers. However, the capacity of such models to realise this potential is subject to both the local context in which they are implemented, such as the pre-existing relationships between contractual partners, but also the wider institutional context, which is still a largely hierarchical system in which individual organisations remain accountable for their individual performance.

8

The changing public health system: an examination of the new commissioning infrastructure

*Stephen Peckham, Anna Coleman, Erica Gadsby,
Julia Segar, Neil Perkins and Donna Bramwell*

Introduction

The wide-ranging reforms made to health and care systems in England, as part of the HSCA 2012, created an enormous shakeup of the way the public health function is delivered. Key public health responsibilities were transferred from the NHS to local government councils. In addition, PHE was established as the national agency for public health.

This chapter examines what these changes have meant for the commissioning of services to improve population health. Commissioning in relation to the health improvement function refers to the strategic planning and purchasing of services that could include smoking cessation, weight management and drug and alcohol services, public health services for children and young people, comprehensive sexual health services and campaigns, dental public health services and services to prevent cancer and long-term conditions.

The political backdrop

The government's goal was to develop a 'public health service that achieves excellent results, unleashing innovation and liberating professional leadership' (Department of Health, 2010b). There were a number of important themes demonstrated in the structural changes. First, they represented an attempt to enhance democratic accountability and challenge the old 'command and control' model. Within the wider context of the localism agenda, the relocation of public health functions was an attempt to ensure that local people made local decisions to improve the health of local populations. Second, the government was attempting to shift the focus from processes onto outcomes. A comprehensive set of indicators were developed within a 'public health outcomes framework', against which local public health systems would be assessed. This would enable transparency and an element of comparability between different local areas. Third, there was an attempt to take a 'different' (though not new) approach to public health – one that takes a 'life course' perspective, and that places importance on wider determinants of health, particularly in relation to people's socioeconomic contexts. Fourth, there was a focus on ensuring that decisions are based on the best possible evidence of what works – a key role for PHE. Fifth, there was an emphasis on efficiency, particularly with regard to being 'joined up' and streamlined. And finally, consistent with wider policy, there was a general push towards commissioning, and lead organisations being solely commissioning organisations.

In this context, the shift of public health functions into local government made inherent sense. It stood to create opportunities for public health staff to work across a wider front, for example with those locally responsible for leisure, planning and environmental health (Stopforth, 2014; Association of Directors of Public Health, 2015;). It was also a move that chimed with national and international research and policy that continued to emphasise environmental and economic determinants of health (Baum, 2008; Campbell, 2010; Marmot, 2010). However, the shift would be far from easy.

Some stakeholders opposed the notion of taking public health out of the NHS. Support for and opposition against such a move have been rehearsed in long-running debates since long before 1974, when public health duties were removed from local councils and the historic position of local Medical Officer of Health was abolished (Gorsky et al, 2014). These debates reflect different emphases on individual versus collective approaches to public health, and different emphases on prevention versus the planning and management of health provision for existing health problems (Berridge et al, 2011). They reflect tensions too around how public health should be defined – for instance, whether it is a medical speciality, a multidisciplinary speciality or 'everybody's business' (Griffiths et al, 2005) and the tension between public or population health as political action as described by Rudolf Virchow in the nineteenth century (Griffiths et al, 2005) or as a professional (particularly medical) specialism (Berridge et al, 2011). Unfortunately, as noted in an Institute of Medicine report (2002), there is so little evidence concerning the optimal structure and operation of public health delivery systems that arguments remain contested, questions remain unanswered, and policy makers have little on which to base their decisions.

Many stakeholders supported the shift to local councils in principle, but expressed a wide range of concerns prior to and during the reforms. Many issues were raised by expert witnesses to the Local Government and Communities Committee of the House of Commons in 2012 about structural capacity, autonomy of public health specialists, and resources (Riches et al, 2015). A survey by the Faculty of Public Health of its membership in 2014 also identified concerns among public health professionals about whether the move would affect their professional status and the public health infrastructure and resourcing (Lambert and Sowden, 2016).

Commissioning public health – then and now

Prior to the reforms in England, PCTs were the NHS bodies responsible for commissioning most health services, including for population health improvement and ill-health prevention (Marks et al, 2011). Until 2011, they also directly managed the vast majority of NHS CHS, such as district nursing, health visiting and children's services. Public health specialists within PCTs provided a lead role in developing strategies for meeting local health needs. They also provided specialist clinical and public health advice to inform PCT commissioning. Whilst they often worked closely with local councils, funding remained predominantly from NHS sources. Directors of Public Health (DsPH) were key PCT Board members and could make executive decisions about public health investments (Marks et al, 2010, 2011).

In 2013, as public health teams transferred to local councils, PCTs were abolished and replaced by CCGs. At the same time, a public health budget was created, separate from that managed through NHSE for healthcare. This budget is decided by the DHSC and managed by PHE. PHE funds public health activity either through allocations to councils, by commissioning services via NHSE, or by commissioning or providing services itself. Local councils now commission or provide most locally delivered public health activities although most clinical interventions (for example, preventive medication) are still delivered within the NHS, especially general practice.

Local councils in the UK provide a wide range of services, including social care, children's services, housing, leisure, parks and planning. The structure of local government in England is complex: there are 125 unitary councils that provide the full range of services, and there are 27 areas where the services are split between upper-tier county councils (taking responsibility for social care, education, transportation and strategic planning), and smaller district councils (covering, for example, housing, leisure, environmental health and planning). All of these councils are run by elected councillors, usually affiliated to a political party, who represent and engage their local population, make key decisions, contribute to policy/strategy review and development, and conduct overview and scrutiny roles. Whilst there is a complex web of legislation and statutory powers and responsibilities governing them (Gains et al, 2004), councils have a great deal of freedom to innovate. Local government has been described as a 'networked polity', adopting partnership and new forms of accountability at a local level (Skelcher and Torfing, 2000; Rhodes, 2007; Sullivan, 2007; Durose et al, 2009). All councils work with a wide range of local partners.

DsPH in councils continue to be involved in making decisions about public health services and expenditure, but elected members are responsible for all decisions, within a political framework. Councils are accountable to PHE for the appropriate use of the public health grant, but to their electorates for delivering outcomes. DsPH like all council officers, are responsible for making sure council policy is carried out.

The HSCA also introduced HWBs as statutory subcommittees of local councils. These boards were intended to bring together the key NHS, public health and social care leaders in each local council area to work together to coordinate commissioning of their services. HWBs are outlined in more detail in Chapter 2.

Research in a changing landscape: The PHOENIX study

PHOENIX (Public Health and Obesity in England – the New Infrastructure eXamined) was one of PRUComm's core research projects. It was a three-year project, starting in April 2013 – just as the new structures described on pages 125–126 were formally launched (though many had operated in shadow form prior to this, and some public health teams had transferred to their local councils up to a year previously). The research examined the development of the reformed public health system in England, and the impact of structural changes on the functioning of the public health system and on the approaches taken to improving the public's health. One of the objectives of the study was to examine approaches taken to commissioning within the new system, using obesity as a focal topic.

The study employed multiple methods to examine key issues at a national level, and to further explore those in local case studies. It began with a scoping review (Gadsby et al, 2014) that included an analysis of policy documents and responses to the reforms from key stakeholders (reported in Riches et al, 2015), to develop a picture of how the new structures were developing and what the key concerns were. Demographic and other data on all 152 upper-tier and unitary local councils in England were collated, which enabled the purposive selection of local councils for the case study research, conducted from March 2014 to September 2015 in five areas. The five selected areas encompassed 13 different councils, including unitary, upper-tier and a sample of lower-tier (district) councils, some of which had a variety of different sharing arrangements. They were diverse in terms of a range of characteristics, including council size, urban or rural location, sociodemographic and economic circumstances, obesity prevalence and political control. This enabled an examination of multiple perspectives and inter- and intra-organisational relationships in a variety of settings.

The case study approach was ideal for capturing the 'lived reality' (Hodkinson and Hodkinson 2001) in the varied sites in a flexible, in-depth and iterative way. Within the sites, PRUComm researchers conducted 103 semi-structured interviews with: 36 council public health staff; 18 elected members; 25 council non-public health staff; 13 provider organisation staff; 6 CCG staff and 3 other staff at regional levels. Fifteen meetings were observed, and a wide range of documentary evidence was collated to enrich understanding of the situation in the case study areas.

To supplement the case study work, a small number of interviews were conducted outside of the case study areas, particularly to explore national- and regional-level issues and relationships with/within PHE. To develop a national view of changes, two web-based questionnaire surveys were conducted, of all DsPH and councillors with a lead responsibility for public health, in all 152 upper-tier and unitary councils. These surveys were undertaken in summer 2014 and autumn 2015 (see Jenkins et al, 2016: for a description of survey methods and a detailed analysis of the first survey). They were focused on the organisation and management of public health teams both within and between councils, lines of communication, budgetary responsibility and managerial accountability, and how well the public health team was functioning and having influence across the council. They also asked about wider relationships, for example with PHE, HWBs and CCGs.

Within the PHOENIX research, commissioning was considered as one of the broad aspects of public health activity – alongside supporting clinical commissioning in CCGs, leading on health protection, and working across the range of the council's business to influence decisions for the benefit of the local population's health. The research set out to examine the context for commissioning, the people/organisations involved in commissioning activities, the processes involved, and any evidence of things changing. It sits alongside other published work, much of which reflected, retrospectively, on the progress and impact of the reforms. This included a House of Commons Health Committee inquiry on public health post-2013, launched October 2015, which raised some important issues related to the structures, organisation, funding and delivery of public health following the reforms (House of Commons Health Committee, 2015).

Results

The new context for commissioning

The transfer of public health staff and resources into local councils from PCTs was far from straightforward, and often accompanied other system reorganisations. Local councils were given the freedom to organise their incoming public health teams in any number of ways. This raised concerns from some commentators about the capacity and autonomy of DsPH within local bureaucracies that might make them subordinate to other officials (House of Commons Health Committee, 2014). This research, like others (Department of Health, 2012a, 2012b), found considerable variation across the country with regard to the 'location' of the public health team and its director within the structure and hierarchy of the council. Within councils, DsPH sit alongside, or sometimes under, other directors who are often presiding over directorates that are far more significant in terms of staffing and budget. Also, elected members in councils have an important political and corporate leadership role across the system. The strength and position of the public health team, and their skills in working with elected members are, therefore, very important.

The transfer process fragmented public health teams. For instance, in many cases, staff groups were dispersed or responsibilities were split. In one case study area, staff in a PCT were separated into a council public health team, into one of three CCGs, or into a provider trust.

In another, a children's public health commissioner, formerly in the children's joint commissioning team in the PCT with commissioning responsibilities for the whole of the 0–19 pathway, was transferred to a council team. Her former commissioning responsibilities were split amongst different organisations, and she was now responsible only for certain elements of the healthy child programme. She explained the resulting confusion: "It has caused fragmentation of the system and certainly for the 0–19 pathway or services for children, you know, the health services for children. It has meant that different parts of the system are now responsible for commissioning different elements of it ... which is challenging" (Senior Public Health Commissioner, Council, Site B). This fragmentation also had implications for the sharing of information between health and council commissioners, which this officer described as being "much more difficult for us now".

Some public health staff chose to join PHE or NHSE, and some became part of new commissioning support organisations. There was much confusion over where staff should be transferred to (sometimes depending on the proportion of their time spent on service commissioning versus service provision), and around the organisation of budgets. There were instances where this tested relationships between councils and CCGs.

Public health staff, responsibilities and resources were transferred to local councils at a time of unprecedented cuts to local government budgets (The Centre for Local Economic Strategies, 2014). These cuts precipitated ongoing organisational restructuring within councils which sought to streamline departmental structures and reduce staffing costs. Individual councils, while generally adopting cost-cutting measures, approached organisational restructuring in different ways, including internal reorganisation and in some cases function sharing with neighbouring councils.

With the freedom to organise public health in different ways, it was not surprising that a range of different organisational models for public health in local councils emerged. The PHOENIX survey conducted in autumn 2015 found that about a quarter of the public health teams were distinct public health directorates; half were sections of another directorate; and the rest represented a wide range of structures including merged, distributed and mixed models. In some cases, DsPH were shared by councils but with different degrees of coordination between the public health teams in the collaborating councils, and involving complex governance arrangements. Such arrangements were often driven by the existence of established joint operational structures for other areas of local council responsibilities.

Changes in decision-making processes were as important as changes in organisational structure. The PHOENIX surveys found that DsPH had different levels of access to key council decision-making bodies. For example, only around half were members of the council's most senior corporate management team. Just under half said they were managerially responsible to the council's chief executive; the remainder were managed by a range of other directorate heads. Consequently, DsPH were less central to decisions about public health investments, and were not always in the best place for strategic influence in the council. This is consistent with the government's desire to increase local democratic accountability for public health – with the idea that elected members have a close connection to and strong engagement with their local populations, and are therefore better able to make decisions that are driven by local need.

However, many public health services have little popular appeal, and their outcomes (particularly in relation to improved population health and wellbeing) are far from immediate. Perceptions regarding the severity of public health issues, where responsibility lies, and who is affected, are likely to vary considerably. The aetiology of many public health issues encompasses strong moral dimensions, and ethical issues and dilemmas often arise. In making DsPH less central to public health decision making, it is possible that decisions may become more politically influenced than informed by evidence (Marks et al, 2015; Kneale et al, 2017). However, it is also possible that a wider understanding of what constitutes evidence is being developed within the local council setting, with a shift away from a hierarchy of scientific evidence and towards more qualitative evidence or consensus opinions, perhaps elicited through community-based participatory research. The relationship between evidence and power might need to be better understood by PHE to know how to support public health decision making and an appropriate use of evidence (Parkhurst and Abeysinghe, 2016).

Commissioning processes and people involved

Decision making within councils is quite different to that in the now extinct PCTs. The governance structures of PCTs were less democratic as the governing board consisted of executive directors (including the DPH) and appointed lay non-executives. This resulted in more executive power for DsPH. In councils, however, decisions about how to spend public health money are subject to a greater range of decision makers and wider consultation, both across the council and amongst the public, than before. The PHOENIX research found that elected members influenced the priorities and actions of the public health team in both overt and implicit ways. Of the 38 councillors who responded to the question in 2015, 45 per cent said they felt always able, and 47 per cent said they were quite often able to influence the priorities of the public health team. The case studies showed how this influence might operate more subtly, perhaps according to the ideologies and interests of the elected member, or the politics of the council. For instance, in one Conservative-led council, the elected member explained that he would have a very difficult job persuading his cabinet to significantly increase spending on smoking cessation: "They're not particularly interested in it, they think … 'oh well if people smoke themselves silly, let them smoke themselves silly'" (Elected member, County Council).

Compared with the NHS, local councils take different approaches to prioritisation and commissioning, influenced in part by over 15 years of implementing 'Best Value'.[1] The processes of commissioning (and new procurement laws) within a council have had to be learned by incoming public health staff. At the same time, public health staff have tried to educate councillors in public health commissioning. In the case study sites, several commissioning officers who had worked within councils prior to the reforms (for example, in adult or children's social care directorates) and who moved, following the reforms, into the public health teams, talked about differences they observed in how commissioning was done. One, referring to her incoming public health colleagues, said that there was a complete lack of understanding about local council-style commissioning and business processes and the fact that local council commissioners had many years' experience. Another talked about the differences between commissioning in PCTs and commissioning in the councils. She explained: "public health has commissioning responsibilities now in a way that they didn't in the old PCT". She described commissioning in the former PCTs as comparatively less "robust", with less accountability, and less scrutiny of performance and outcomes data, reflecting on the fact that: "there's much stronger scrutiny in local government and that's all areas of business and it's something that we've had to really work with our providers in NHS specifically around understanding" (Commissioner,

---

[1]   The Duty of Best Value makes clear that councils should consider overall value – including social value – when looking at service provision. Under the general Duty of Best Value, local authorities should 'make arrangements to secure continuous improvement in the way in which its functions are exercised, having regard to a combination of economy, efficiency and effectiveness', www.gov.uk/government/publications/best-value-statutory-guidance--4

Council, Site A). This suggests that the government's desire to focus more on efficiency and outcomes might be more easily realised in the new context of public health commissioning.

From the point of view of providers, however, the sometimes rather narrow outcomes-based scrutiny that services were now subjected to was not always appropriate for complex public health interventions. For instance, the provider of a range of obesity prevention services in one of the case study areas complained that the focus on outcomes in terms of body mass index reductions belied the fact that most of their time and resources were spent on engaging communities and developing relationships with schools and others. The more proximal outcomes of this type of activity, however, are impossible to measure.

Having a distinct public health grant for the first time enabled DsPH to take a different approach – a more strategic approach – to the allocation of the public health budget. A public health officer in one of the sites described how, in the PCT, they were sometimes left 'scrabbling' around for funds, when public health priorities and PCT priorities were not always well matched. However, with a ring-fenced budget, they were able to plan how best to match spending against their local priorities. The leader of a county council in one of the case study sites explained how they were prepared to completely shake up the way in which the public health grant was spent: "We've got to start at reviewing; is that delivering to the right priorities or not? Is it value for money or not? And what should we stop doing and what should we start doing?" Indeed, councillors in all of the case study sites demanded this process of wholescale service reviews for specific areas, such as obesity. For public health officers, this sometimes gave them the freedom to pursue quite different approaches.

Decision making across the local system following the reforms was intended to be more coordinated. However, with commissioning responsibilities now fragmented between NHSE, PHE, local councils and CCGs, the research found that coordination was proving to be difficult. Moreover, the lack of clarity about responsibilities sometimes led to delays in the commissioning of services, and/or tensions in the relationships between organisations. Commissioning across an obesity pathway, for instance, involves councils (for broad obesity prevention and non-intensive weight management services), CCGs (for specialist obesity services) and NHSE (bariatric services) (Department of Health, 2013a; NICE, 2014). Across England, there are significant gaps in this pathway, with a particular lack of specialist obesity services (Hughes, 2015; Public Health England, 2015). Following the reforms, there was a great deal of confusion about whose responsibility it was to commission these services.

It is clear that, as with many public health interventions, if weight management and obesity prevention services are to achieve their objectives, primary and community care providers play a vital role. The presence, absence, type and success of health improvement services commissioned by councils have important implications for NHS work. However, there is now a greater disconnect between public health officers and NHS commissioners. In the PHOENIX surveys of DsPH, nearly half of those responding said they felt 'less able' to influence local CCGs than before the reforms. In the case study sites, there was limited evidence of meaningful engagement between public health teams and CCGs. A HWB Chair in one of the sites felt that CCGs had become disengaged from public health, and that they now had to persuade the CCG that public health is everybody's business, not just the responsibility of the local council. He commented that "they see public health as a separate entity at the moment, and not part of an integrated health economy" (Chair HWB, Council, Site C).

Although HWBs were meant to be the mechanism for coordinating commissioning across NHS, social care and public health at the strategic level, the PHOENIX survey suggested that the new Boards were limited in their impact and influence. Just less than half of the DsPH in the 2015 survey felt the HWB was 'definitely' instrumental in identifying the main health and wellbeing priorities (48 per cent, $N = 65$), and that HWBs 'definitely' strengthened relationships between commissioning organisations (45 per cent, $N = 65$). Less than 5 per cent felt that the HWB was 'definitely' making difficult decisions, and only about a quarter felt that it had 'definitely' begun to address the wider determinants of health.

A further complication with coordinating across the system and addressing wider determinants is that in two-tier councils many of the functions that public health are expected to work across are based in multiple lower-tier district councils. Public health officers must therefore build relationships with a greater number of different organisations, all with their own priorities and ideas. In addition, these district councils often have a limited voice on HWBs. It is perhaps for this reason, in part, that some HWBs were not seen to be significantly engaging with the public health agenda. However, there were also other distractions for HWBs, particularly in the emphasis on integration and the Better Care Fund – highlighted by some case study interviewees as another reason for less focus on public health.

Commissioned services: what has changed?

Whilst the context and processes of public health commissioning have changed dramatically, it is important to reflect on whether this leads to any significant change in the type, quantity or balance of services commissioned. One of the expectations of the reforms might have been that public health teams, in their new setting, might take quite different approaches to health improvement. One difference in approach might be to commission less in the way of services (particularly, for instance, individual behaviour change services), and do more in the way of creating structural or procedural changes that support health improvement across policy areas and over the long term (for instance, by influencing planning decisions or transport strategies). For this type of work, staffing is likely to be the most important resource (Local Government Association, 2016), so capacity within the public health team is important. Additionally, public health resources might be used to invest in those council activities that can have a positive impact on the wellbeing and health of people who live, work and learn in the local area.

Whilst it will take time for the full impact of the reforms in terms of changes to commissioned services to be realised, the PHOENIX research suggested that, even in the initial few years, public health commissioning was beginning to change on a number of levels. Firstly, money was being used in different ways. For example, 89 per cent of DPH respondents to the 2015 survey said that the public health budget had been used to invest in other council departments in the previous 12 months. Most DsPH felt the public health budget was expected to contribute to the overall savings that councils needed to make. Many seemed reconciled that the budget would now be used to fund other services – in many cases, services that would have been cut (for example, children's centres) had public health funding not been available. However, such investments might in fact make important contributions to health improvement. Public Health Officers in the case studies talked about the opportunities presented, in terms of embedding public health activities and objectives within other council services and providing more joined-up ways of thinking and working.

Secondly, there were many changes being made to the commissioning of health improvement services (see Figure 8.1). The move to local government prompted Public Health Commissioners to look at services and contracts anew. In addition, councils tended towards shorter contracts and more frequent retendering of services than the NHS. All the respondents had started the process of retendering within two years.

Figure 8.1: Has your local authority made any changes to services commissioned under the ring-fenced public health budget? (2015 and 2014 DPH national surveys)

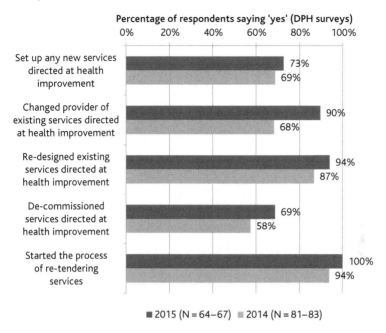

Note: the figure shows responses to several questions, and a range in *N* gives the maximum and minimum number answering each of the questions.

But nearly three-quarters of responding councils had set up new services, and most had changed the provider of existing services and redesigned existing services. About two-thirds of councils had decommissioned services directed at health improvement in the previous 12 months. In the case study sites, extensive commissioning changes sometimes occurred as a result of changes in local area arrangements – for instance, where several areas (former PCTs) were brought together into one (council). Other commissioning changes, however, were as a result of service reviews that were very critical of service outcomes.

A more recent analysis of council spending on public health by the King's Fund (Buck, 2018) showed that spending on public health has changed little from 2013–14 to 2017–18 (forecast), although the amount is likely to be worth 4–5 per cent less and needs to cover a population about 3 per cent larger (based on Office for National Statistics forecasts). Looking at major categories of spending between 2015–16 and 2016–17, there were decreases in most categories, with the biggest being in sexual health services (promotion, prevention and advice, cut by over 30 per cent), wider tobacco control (over 30 per cent), stop smoking services and interventions, and specialist drug and alcohol misuse services for children and young people (approximately 15 per cent). It is important to note that budget is not a good indication of quality or outcomes. For example, despite the significant cuts in budget, there has been a 13 per cent increase in the number of attendances for sexual health services from 2013 to 2017. Similarly, the total number of sexual health screens (tests for common sexual health diseases) increased by 18 per cent over the same time period. Diagnoses, meanwhile, remain relatively static (Public Health England, 2018).

The budgets are clearly under increasing pressure. In a report on funding for public health in the UK, the British Medical Association (2017) pointed out that public health advice to NHS commissioners is one of the functions most affected by cuts to the budgets, and that this is likely to discourage strong working relationships between local councils and CCGs. It also has the potential to reduce the public health advice being used to support the development of ongoing plans for integrating health and care.

The PHOENIX surveys asked for more information about changes that were being made to obesity commissioning. DsPH commented that they wanted to move away from ineffective schemes, increase their focus on children, use new providers and create a more integrated pathway. All these changes resulted in different commissioned service profiles, as well as insecurity in the provider landscape.

The increasing emphasis on commissioning as an activity also had important consequences for the structure of public health teams in local councils. During the period of the PHOENIX research, there was a significant change in the size and profile of the public health teams responsible for commissioning health improvement services. Over a quarter of DsPH reported changes to the size and composition of their public health team, with fewer public health specialists, more business managers/commissioning support staff, and more 'other' staff (not falling into the DPH, specialist, analyst or commissioning support categories). In the case study sites, Public Health Officers talked of the need to address skill gaps within their team in response to working in the new environment. In one site, for instance, the public health commissioning team (made up of non-public health specialists) had been significantly bolstered. The team of public health specialists had been correspondingly reduced. This might affect the extent to which public health teams can create structural or procedural changes that support health improvement across all council areas.

It was not easy to tell, at the time of the research whether these observed changes had resulted in a significantly different set of activities being commissioned. However, there were early signs of some general shifts occurring. In three of the case study areas, a shift towards the commissioning of more holistic 'healthy lifestyle' services was observed, bringing together weight management, smoking cessation, alcohol reduction, sexual health services and so on – perhaps as part of an attempt to save money and consolidate services. In two councils, there was a shift (at least in rhetoric) towards 'whole council' approaches, for instance, where they were seeking to address a broader range of factors influencing obesity, particularly by working across council departments. A greater recognition of public health objectives and expected outcomes was witnessed in a wider range of council services as a result of public health investment. And public health staff were seen working hard to influence the wider workforce. Particularly during the transition phase, as public health bodies were settling into their new homes, a number of programmes including learning events, information sharing, and engagement events were targeted at elected members and non-public health officers across the council.

Discussion

The reforms aimed to bring about changes in five broad dimensions: enhancing local decision making and accountability for local population health improvement; bringing opportunities to effectively tackle wider determinants of health; emphasising outcomes-driven activity; ensuring decisions and activities are driven by what works; and improving efficiency by creating a system that is more streamlined and joined up. Work by PRUComm and others, described in this chapter, suggests a very mixed degree of success in achieving these aims.

Public health decision making in the new context of local councils is undoubtedly very different; DsPH are influencers, rather than executive-level decision makers, and decisions are made within a more political framework, with elected members being ultimately accountable. Public health decisions are open to a different type and a more intense degree of scrutiny in councils, and are likely to be influenced by a wider range of factors and voices. This could help to achieve (in theory) the desired aim of enhancing local accountability and achieving context-relevant action driven by local need, but this will be dependent in part on the level and type of citizen engagement. Few local public health decisions are likely to be vote winners, and they will often depend on an in-depth understanding of moral and ethical implications and trade-offs. Whilst local councils are historically better at citizen engagement than the NHS (Ruane, 2014), to achieve local public health decisions made by local people, for local people, councils will probably need to ensure they are doing more to promote deliberative inclusive approaches.

Whilst the potential for local democratic accountability may have been enhanced, there is also a need for formal state-driven accountability. There were inherent weaknesses in the accountability framework within the post-reform health system – local councils were afforded considerable discretion in how they interpreted the full and detailed scope of their new function and services (Peckham et al, 2016). They have a great deal of independence as democratic organisations, and very few conditions were set on the spending of public health grants. This means that public health decision making, and the way in which the budget is spent, is now less amenable to central government control (Gadsby et al, 2017b).

The research highlighted the diversity in structures, roles and responsibilities already being created between different councils. This is likely to continue. There also seems to be more opportunity for variation across the country in what activity is commissioned, and in who provides it (as well as how, where and to whom). Whilst this is not necessarily a bad thing – difference in local need ought to imply difference in local priorities and provision – the mechanisms by which local councils can be compared, challenged and held to account have not been fully considered, and it is difficult to assess the contributions local councils are making towards improvements in prevention and public health. Whilst the freedom to innovate might create an excellent space for new public health approaches to flourish, it is vital that learning is generated from these innovations – this will require an emphasis on evaluation, and appropriate funding and expertise.

As part of the new decision-making framework, public health staff have had to get used to a new level of bureaucracy, and have had to learn new skills, for instance in political advocacy. Elected members may be less influenced by scientific evidence of what works, and more by the council's ideological, historical and political values and preferences. The House of Commons Health Committee (2016), in its report on public health post-2013, described this as the tension between politics and evidence. The notion of what evidence counts as 'good' evidence in this context may be changing, and this is a debate worth stimulating. There is an increasing call for more discussion about the reasoning and evidence necessary to meet contemporary public health challenges (Rutter et al, 2017; The Health Foundation, 2018). However, it is a development that will need to be supported by PHE and the wider research and knowledge translation communities.

Commissioning in local councils has historically become 'part of the core repertoire of modern strategic management' – it carries an implication of change, with the aspiration of service reform, redesign or reconfiguration (Bennett, 2015: 3). This contrasts with the history of commissioning in the NHS, where there has been a tendency for commissioners and providers to have more permanent relationships. The PHOENIX research highlighted that there was a great deal of change in service redesign and decommissioning following the transfer in 2013. In addition, there were changes in public health team profiles, which reflected a greater emphasis on commissioning skills and a decreased emphasis on specialist public health skills. There were signs that in the councils, decisions were being scrutinised more in terms of the outcomes they bring about, and their value for money (in the context of ever-decreasing budgets), which is likely good news from a government's point of view. However, from the providers' point of view, this meant uncertainty and sometimes an oversimplification of the complexity of generating population health improvements, which are multi-causal and long term in nature. The focus on outcomes lends itself to simple, linear, causal models. Rutter and colleagues (2017) argue, however, that a shift in thinking is required in order to consider health improvements as outcomes that result from a multitude of interdependent elements. Local councils will require support to ensure they judge public health actions on the right terms and over the right timeframes.

One of the clear opportunities presented by shifting public health into local councils was the potential for public health staff to work in different ways, to create changes that support health improvement across other policy areas. It was certainly seen that the public health budget was being invested in other parts of councils, and qualitative evidence suggested that this was sometimes positive, enabling public health outcomes to be embedded in other council activity. However, it was also clear that it was sometimes a response to overall severe council budget cuts; this was interpreted by some commentators as 'budget raiding' (Iacobucci, 2014). There were examples in the case study sites of small steps towards creating 'public health councils'. There are other examples too, such as those described by the Local Government Association (2018), that illustrate ways in which public health teams have seized opportunities to work with communities and support inclusive growth, good housing and jobs policy within their councils. However, there were such examples prior to the reforms, and it is not clear whether a relocation of public health into councils was necessary for such examples to proliferate, or whether the benefits of the relocation outweigh the costs. Moreover, such action requires staff capacity; evidence suggests that public health staff are increasingly being lost from each subsequent council restructure.

The considerable upheaval initiated by the transfer of public health into local councils, and continued by the almost constant reorganisations necessitated by budget cuts, has arguably been one of the greatest 'costs' of the reforms in public health. The process of transition was difficult and confusing for many; some of this confusion might have been anticipated and mitigated against with improved planning, predicated on a better understanding of local councils and the way they work. In particular, two-tier councils and the role of district councils in health improvement were largely ignored in the run-up to the transition. The reforms simplified some aspects of the public health function, for example by bringing public health specialists from over 70 former organisations into the new PHE, and by identifying a specific public health grant. However, it also brought confusion and fragmentation, for example where commissioning for certain services was divided between different bodies. Boundary issues also brought confusion with regard to national system-level leadership, with the relationships between the DH, PHE and NHSE being unclear (House of Commons Health Committee, 2016).

As the new system was taking shape, commissioners found that they often lacked guidance and clarity from government. In particular, public health officers expressed the need for more timely information, for instance regarding responsibilities for commissioning across the fragmented system, or how the in-year budget cuts would be implemented (Department of Health, 2015). In the absence of detailed information, public health teams were sometimes forced to make commissioning decisions based more on expediency than on need. In the new system, the DHSC takes a strategic leadership role, improving people's health and wellbeing through its stewardship of the public health system (Department of Health, 2010b). However, there are grounds for concern about the commitment at national level to population-wide health improvement. Geographical inequalities in life expectancy have increased since 2010, reversing a decline that was seen during the period of the English health inequalities strategy (1997 to 2010) (Barr et al, 2017).

A further 'cost' of the reforms is the distance they have created between public health staff and NHS commissioners. Whilst local council public health teams are mandated to provide public health advice to NHS commissioners, this role is threatened by a shortage of (particularly consultant-grade) public health staff, as well as access to data and capacity to analyse it (House of Commons Health Committee, 2016). The programme of upheaval that the NHS has been subject to has added further complications. Ultimately, the separation between NHS, public health and social care budgets and commissioning responsibility in the long term is unlikely to facilitate a coordinated approach to health and wellbeing improvement. HWBs – charged with ensuring strategic direction across organisations – have not lived up to the expectations placed upon them (Coleman et al, 2014). Efforts at a local level to work together to improve health and wellbeing and reduce health inequalities have been stymied by the ongoing efforts to redesign ways of delivering care in response to the changing needs of patients, and in response to the need to bridge a financial gap estimated to be £22 billion by 2020–21 (Ham, 2017). Public health specialists have not been central to the development of STPs, and illness prevention has taken second place to a focus on the quality and sustainability of health and social care services (Alderwick et al, 2016).

In reflecting on the return of public health to local government Gorsky and colleagues (2014: 550) noted that 'It will be important to consider how to maximize the impact of the statutory DsPH annual reports within a democratically elected organization, while learning to maximize the use of local consultation strategies and new communication approaches to engage local public and political support'. In particular they point to the DPH's statutory duty to address inequalities in access and outcomes. This reflects the importance of the Marmot review and its influence on proposals to broaden the public health perspectives of local government. However, as Gorsky and colleagues (2014) and Marks and colleagues (2015) note, local councils need to develop clear public health visions which prioritise tackling wider societal causes of poor health and inequality at a time when local government is itself under extreme stress, within a broader context that is framed by an 'enduring political rhetoric which focuses on changing "individual behaviour" and defends personal choices over regulation and "nannying"' (Gorsky et al, 2014: 550). There also needs to be an acceptance that there will be local variation of public health services – given variation is an obvious consequence of local governance. However, as Masters and colleagues (2017) show, national programmes to address public health issues can result in significant returns on investment and there remains a clear need for government action on many aspects of public health. Even after five years, the responsibilities, balance of action and approaches to local public health are still very much in a state of flux.

9

Conclusion

Pauline Allen, Kath Checkland, Stephen Peckham and Valerie Moran

The period since the passing of the HSCA 2012 has been one of change and disruption for the NHS and at the time of writing in 2019 it seems unlikely that this turbulence will diminish in the near future. While the LTP (NHS England and NHS Improvement, 2019) published in January 2019 provides some indication of the future direction of commissioning, the lack of specific detail and guidance leaves the Plan open to interpretation. The main thrust of the LTP is to increase the emphasis on collaboration and integration at local level at the expense of competition, but its provisions about commissioning itself are not clear. The structural changes introduced by the HSCA 2012 pursuant to the twin policies of increasing clinical involvement in commissioning and accelerating market forces have had large effects on the practice of commissioning across the NHS. The government also emphasised the need for local freedoms to determine how services should be delivered in relation to the choices and needs of patients and greater public and democratic accountability (Department of Health, 2010a). In addition, while the focus of less attention, the shift of public health from the NHS to LAs discussed in Chapter 8 has also had a profound effect on the commissioning and delivery of services. The broad range of PRUComm's research projects has revealed a series of common themes, which are also found in other research on developments during this period.

As highlighted in previous chapters, since the introduction of changes following the HSCA 2012 there has been a large increase in the complexity of health system governance. The number of bodies undertaking commissioning has increased in two ways: NHSE, PHE and LAs all have a role in commissioning aspects of health care, in addition to CCGs, which were the successor to PCTs; moreover, CCGs are smaller organisations than PCTs so there are many more of them. While the shift to CCGs and LA commissioning appears to fit with the White Paper's language of localism and decentralisation, freeing local commissioners from central control, the reality has been somewhat more mixed. Clearly the national commissioning roles of NHSE and PHE involved the centralisation of some activities previously undertaken by PCTs but commissioning responsibilities have remained fluid. Since 2013, some responsibilities have been passed from NHSE to CCGs and LAs (for example, health visiting to LAs and some responsibility for primary care commissioning to CCGs).

As well as the proliferation of commissioning organisations, there has also been an increase in the number of other NHS organisations required to regulate the complex system: initially Monitor, as economic regulator, was joined by the TDA (they have since been merged into NHSI); NHSE was established to be responsible for commissioning at national level; and the CQC was established in 2008 as the main regulator of quality. Other local organisations known as clinical senates were also introduced in order to give clinicians other than GPs a voice – although their role is purely advisory. The effect of this increase in complexity in the governance of the NHS has been wide-ranging. As a result, local autonomy is severely limited and the aspirations set out in the White Paper to deliver freedom from government control and greater accountability to patients and greater democratic legitimacy (Department of Health, 2010a) have not been realised to any significant degree. Overall the picture has been one of the delegation of responsibility for local planning and delivery to local organisations with increasing central control over outcomes and regulation (Checkland et al, 2017).

However, the fragmentation of commissioning roles has been damaging to the planning and delivery of services which are subject to several commissioning regimes (Gadsby et al, 2017a; Checkland et al, 2018c). It was envisaged that greater coordination of commissioning at a local level would be achieved through HWBs but on the whole, these have not played a significant role in coordination or setting strategic direction and have increasingly been focused on issues related to the Better Care Fund (Peckham et al, 2015; Coleman et al, 2016). In their current form, HWBs have generally been unable to take on these roles as they have little power to hold partners and organisations to account (Hunter et al, 2018). With the establishment of STPs, which have a larger geographical footprint and arguably more traction on the system because of their pivotal role in the centrally defined NHS commissioning structures, there is a question mark over how HWB roles will develop in the future.

One particularly difficult area has been sexual health services because these involve elements of public health preventive action as well as healthcare interventions of various degrees of complexity and expense.

Sexual health services now straddle three types of commissioners: CCGs (for example, for termination of pregnancy), LAs (for example, for sexual health promotion) and NHSE (for example, for HIV treatment) (Hammond et al, 2017). The greater the number of commissioning organisations involved in sexual health, the greater the disruption to services (Checkland et al, 2018c). According to the LTP (NHS England and NHS Improvement, 2019), the government and the NHS will consider future arrangements for the commissioning of sexual health services and whether the NHS should play a stronger role. Similarly, in the research on the public health system problems were found associated with responsibilities for obesity services – especially tier three and whether CCGs or LAs were the relevant funder (Peckham et al, 2015). Not only is there evidence of deterioration in patient outcomes (Checkland et al, 2018c), but the research has also demonstrated that significant effort, and thus opportunity cost, is required from commissioners to 'knit back together' pre-existing systems of service planning and delivery (Checkland et al, 2018c). In a situation where management costs of commissioners have been severely constrained by nationally set CCG management allowances (McDermott et al, 2015), it is unfortunate to be obliged to spend management resources on ameliorating a situation which has deteriorated due to the architecture of the HSCA 2012.

The issue of accountability of commissioners is closely related to the problem of increased complexity of commissioning and system governance. CCGs are stated to be membership organisations whose primary accountability is internally to their GP members. But there are other actors to whom they also owe accountability. The strongest form of accountability would seem to be their hierarchical upwards accountability to NHSE, backed by sanctions and subject to annual assessment. Furthermore, the currency of this accountability is clearly established, encompassing fiscal accountability and programme accountability for the Clinical Commissioning Group Outcomes Indicator Set. The accountability to other external bodies such as HWBs is, by contrast, much weaker, and less clearly defined, with CCGs required to 'give an account', with no associated sanctions.

Accountability to NHSI is more formal, as it is currently empowered to enforce competition and procurement law, although future legislative change could dispense with its competition roles (NHS England and NHS Improvement, 2019). And it is also envisaged that NHSE and NHSI will formally merge. If these changes are made, the main form of accountability for NHS providers and CCGs will be hierarchical – upwards to the merged body. Accountability to the public is a political accountability, focused on the relatively weak notion of 'transparency', with no associated sanctions. Internal accountability is similarly complex, with a mix of mutual and one-way relationships, some accompanied by the ultimate sanction of voting out office holders. General practices are said to be 'held to account' if they transgress the rules of the group, but it is unclear as yet if they could be ejected, as all general practices must be a member of a CCG (Checkland et al, 2013a). The strong hierarchical accountability to NHSE can be at odds with internal accountability to members and external horizontal accountability to other local organisations, such as LAs and members of the public (Checkland et al, 2013a). For example, NHSE has been particularly concerned that CCGs' financial obligations do not exceed their nationally set commissioning budgets, whereas the public and LAs are concerned that sufficient services are available locally (House of Commons Health and Social Care Committee, 2018).

The internal governance structures of CCGs also produce accountability problems for governing bodies when CCGs are involved in commissioning primary care locally. Conflicts of interest have been recognised as an important issue since the inception of CCGs, and is probably the explanation for the role initially given to NHSE to commission primary care. The problem gained renewed attention with the delegation of responsibility for commissioning of primary care to CCGs which started to become national policy in 2015. This policy presents a risk that groups of GPs will commission themselves or their practices to provide services. GPs commissioning primary care face conflicts of interest in the form of self-dealing, similar to those faced by managers in business. A range of corporate governance mechanisms has been devised to prevent corporate managers from engaging in conflicts of interest, most notably the use of independent boards to monitor management on behalf of shareholders. Simply increasing transparency by disclosing a potential conflict of interest is not viewed as an adequate measure to prevent undesirable behaviour in the corporate world. Giving CCGs the responsibility to commission primary care created a structural conflict of interest, which cannot be adequately addressed with governance structures and regulations that stress transparency. Simply disclosing an interest does not prevent GPs and practice managers from influencing discussions about primary care, which may undermine their public stewardship role in respect of commissioning budgets (Moran et al, 2017a).

At the level above individual CCGs, the LTP (NHS England and NHS Improvement, 2019) proposes a new ICS accountability and performance framework to consolidate local accountability measures to improve consistency and comparability. Moreover, ICSs will agree system-wide objectives with the national bodies (or merged body) and be held to account for performance against these objectives with the potential to earn greater financial autonomy based on performance. However, as it is not proposed that ICSs are established as statutory organisations, but instead consist of networks of separate bodies, accountability of ICSs will be hard to achieve in the face of the individual organisations' differing statutory accountabilities, which may conflict with the aims of the ICSs. The LTP (NHS England and NHS Improvement, 2019) has also sought to improve accountability of the NHS at national level by endorsing the continuation of a new national body set up to help inform the writing of the Plan – the NHS Assembly. This body of 50 appointed members is designed to increase the accountability of NHSE and NHSI to patients, the public, clinical staff, NHS local leaders and the third sector, although it does not have any formal powers to sanction NHSE or NHSI.

The complex regulatory structures of the NHS required to police the marketised system introduced by the HSCA 2012 have effects on the efficiency of the system as a whole. As discussed in Chapter 1, theories of institutional economics, and transactions costs in particular, indicate that inappropriate use of market institutional structures, as opposed to integrated hierarchies, can decrease overall efficiency by increasing 'frictional' costs of undertaking transactions. In the case of the post-HSCA 2012 NHS, there are two main interrelated aspects of these costs. First, contracts can be understood as the primary regulatory tool. The making, monitoring and enforcement of multiple contracts between commissioners and a wide range of providers across the NHS incurs substantial transactions costs. These are likely to be higher where non-state for-profit providers of care enter the NHS market, as greater effort will be required to negotiate with new entrants and greater effort should be made to monitor the performance of organisations whose incentives to skimp on quality to increase profits are greater than those of NHS organisations (which cannot distribute profits). Secondly, the procurement regulations set out in the HSCA 2012 and the statutory instrument made pursuant to it, together with the European Union rules on public procurement translated into English legislation concerning public contracts, all have the effect of complicating the procedures for identifying a contracting partner to provide healthcare to NHS patients (see Chapter 6). Complying with these complex procedures required by the regulatory regime have been shown to be resource intensive for both commissioners and providers (Sanderson et al, 2017; Osipovic et al, 2019). Even the additional costs incurred by providers will ultimately be borne by the state, as they will be reflected in the prices charged to the NHS. The LTP (NHS England and NHS Improvement, 2019) suggests legislative change to repeal the specific procurement requirements in the HSCA 2012 and remove the NHS from wholesale inclusion in the PCR 2015. Commissioners would have more freedom to decide when they should use procurement, conditional on a 'best value' test to ensure the optimal outcomes for patients and the public purse. However, it is unclear what criteria would underpin the proposed 'best value' test, and whether these would in fact reduce transactions costs for commissioners.

A further effect of the changes to commissioning introduced by the HSCA 2012 has been on clinicians in primary care. Despite the fact that the research has indicated that they can make a useful contribution to commissioning by CCGs (see Chapter 5), the workload associated with such involvement is substantial, with a potentially damaging effect on the working lives of GPs, who are already under stress from excessive demands on their time (Gibson et al, 2017). This makes the sustainability of the model of GP involvement in CCGs dubious, with few younger GPs indicating any appetite to take on these extra responsibilities (Moran et al, 2017b). This is particularly relevant given other developments affecting general practice such as ICSs and GP federations, and the move towards establishing primary care networks proposed in the LTP. In addition, it was found that maximising the potential for clinicians to beneficially influence commissioning requires skilled management at the local level. In keeping with the theoretical focus upon the local implementation of national policy initiatives, the studies collectively demonstrate the importance of skilled and trusted local managers, who understand the local NHS context, have good relationships across all sectors and, most importantly, understand the history of previous NHS initiatives and are able to mobilise learning from these previous policies (McDermott et al, 2018).

Despite the problems caused by the complexity of the NHS system architecture since 2012, the research also found that system actors find ways to coordinate their activities and protect the system as a whole. In addition to the efforts to knit together commissioning for particular services, such as sexual health mentioned on p 45, it was also found that some actors are adept in reducing the financial risks to the system. An important example is the decision in some places not to use the national tariff to pay for inpatient care, despite the formal pricing rules issued by NHSE (see Chapter 7). Instead, some commissioners and providers have agreed block contract sums, which amount to a set budget, allowing commissioners to fix their financial exposure, rather than the open-ended risk of cost-per-case pricing. Proposed reforms of the payment system indicate a move away from the national tariff towards a 'blended' payment approach for emergency care (NHS England and NHS Improvement, 2018a, 2019). The proposed approach consists of a fixed amount based on expected levels of activity and a volume-related element based on actual activity. Additionally, payment system reform will move funding away from activity-based payments towards more population-based funding. However, volume-related payments for elective care will be retained as appropriate. The LTP also proposes new incentives for improvements in quality but does not specify what these incentives will be, along with reforms to the CQUIN framework (NHS England and NHS Improvement, 2019). This would provide greater stability and encourage joint responsibility between commissioners and providers for managing increases in acute activity. A further example of these attempts to protect the financial position of the local NHS is the observation that not all commissioners use competitive procurement as specified by the HSCA 2012 (see Chapter 6). Instead, forms of cooperation with incumbent NHS providers have been used to reconfigure local services. These have been supported by the use of formal mechanisms such as alliance contracts, which promote cooperation and risk sharing between local organisations (see Chapter 7). The LTP (NHS England and NHS Improvement, 2019) supports the continued use of alliance contracts to support service integration.

Since the publication of the FYFV in 2014, these examples of coordination at local level have been seen to be going with the grain of government policy (at least NHSE, even if the procompetitive legislation has not been amended). Indeed, the later introduction of STPs and then ICSs have further encouraged (and sometimes mandated) a place-based, cooperative approach at local level. This notion of place-based cooperation has been closely linked to the concept of 'integrated care' (House of Commons Health and Social Care Committee, 2018). Integrated care is an enduring concept long predating the focus put on it in recent policies. The problem is that the concept is not clearly defined or understood. As the House of Commons Health and Social Care Committee (2018) pointed out, integration of services is a means to a range of ends in respect of patient experience, outcomes and system efficiency, not an end in itself. In fact, the existing evidence does not support the contention that integrating service delivery always reduces cost. For example, studies of 'hospital at home' services, in which integrated support teams are mobilised to support people at home who might otherwise be admitted to hospital, suggest that, whilst daily costs may be lower, care is generally required for longer, leading to no overall reduction in costs (Munton et al, 2011). Furthermore, studies of multidisciplinary team working (a common manifestation of so-called integrated care) fail to demonstrate significant reductions in admissions or costs (Stokes et al, 2016).

The planning and delivery of local services has also been affected by the cuts in LA budgets – particularly in relation to public health and social care and concerns about the impact on morbidity and mortality (Green et al, 2017; Watkins et al, 2017; Hiam et al, 2018). The increasing necessity to deliver more integrated health and social care services for people with long-term and more complex care needs has sought to highlighted resource issues – especially where the NHS has retained some growth whereas LA budgets have been drastically reduced. In the last two years NHSE has highlighted the need for, and called for, more investment in social care to relieve pressures on the NHS (Illman and Dunhill, 2016). In addition, following initial protection of public health budgets these have been subject to annual reductions since 2015 leading to withdrawal of key prevention services in some areas (Iacobucci, 2016, 2017). Yet at the same time as social care budgets have been cut, LA Adult Social Services Departments have had new responsibilities for prevention placed upon them by the Care Act 2014 (Daly and Westwood, 2017). These funding trends continue to cause uncertainty about the ability of local health and social care systems adequately to address local needs for care.

The LTP provides some indication of how place-based integrated care may develop. The LTP envisions national coverage of ICSs by April 2021, which will develop from STPs. Nevertheless, this leaves some ambiguity about the size of the ICS footprint. ICSs will be expected to work with LAs at 'place' level, which indicates that ICSs may be coterminous with LAs – although how linkage with multiple LAs will be handled is not addressed. Commissioners and providers will share decision making about the funding and delivery of services at the ICS level but decisions relating to contracts and procurement will be reserved for commissioners. In order to support a place-based approach, the LTP specifies that CCGs and NHS Trusts should not improve the financial position of their individual organisations at the expense of the overall system. It is unclear how this will be incentivised or operationalised in practice beyond a system oversight approach, which will review organisational and system objectives together with organisational performance to find system-wide solutions. In particular, the LTP does not provide any detail on a system-wide control total, which would hold an ICS collectively accountable for financial performance. ICSs will also have 'streamlined' commissioning arrangements and it is expected that a single CCG will cover each ICS area. The LTP indicates that CCGs will be 'leaner' and 'more strategic' and will support providers to collaborate with LAs and community organisations. While every ICS will have a Partnership Board representing the constituent organisations, with a non-executive Chair and non-executive representation from CCGs and providers, there is no clear guidance on governance and accountability structures. The LTP only refers once to the role of HWBs, suggesting they should work closely with ICSs. It is likely that HWBs (and indeed LAs) may be sidelined by the new partnership structures envisaged in the LTP. It is already apparent that some ICSs do not include LAs (Brennan, 2019).

Irrespective of how the vision in the LTP is implemented, there will always be a role for planning, and thus a degree of commissioning in the NHS, as a publicly funded system. Strategic decisions need to be made about the allocation of public resources between different services in order to optimise population health and wellbeing. Furthermore, it is necessary to monitor the performance of providers of care and make improvements where care is substandard. Thus, the core activities of commissioning are necessary whether pro-competitive quasi-market aspects of the English NHS are retained or not. If commissioning in its current form will endure remains to be seen. Although it is envisaged that CCGs will continue to merge until there is one CCG for each ICS, detailed specification and monitoring of individual services may be undertaken by other bodies (possibly lead providers of networks of subcontractors or alliance contract parties) in some areas. With the development of primary care networks envisaged in the LTP, the contracting and subcontracting arrangements for primary care services will become more complex. The LTP suggests that primary care networks will be both providers and contractors of GP and some other primary care services, introducing a further layer of 'commissioning' within the local health and social care system. Such networks will themselves need to be held to account, and it is unclear how this might work as CCGs get bigger and reduce their role in local commissioning.

These fundamental tasks of service planning and monitoring are essential to an effective healthcare system, whether they are labelled 'commissioning' or not. The LTP has signposted some of the current organisational trends that have been developing within the NHS since 2012. The fracturing of the NHS landscape caused by the HSCA 2012 has resulted in a significant period of organisational turbulence in the English NHS. This has occurred at a time of increased financial constraint in the NHS and, perhaps more significantly, in LA funding. While not a new concept, integration, both between different health care services and between health and social care, is now a core policy priority but also a locally driven response to the various financial and demand pressures on the health and social care system. Primary care remains central to much of the focus of policy, but with the development of integrated commissioning systems, mergers of CCGs and the development of primary care networks and integrated providers the healthcare landscape remains in a state of flux. There continues to be a lack of clarity about the roles and functions of different organisations and structures and the contract, incentive and accountability processes that are emerging. There also remain significant financial pressures on the health and social care system, with demands for additional resources in the NHS partly met by recent funding allocations but without, as yet, a clear plan for social care funding and with sustained cuts to public health funding which will continue to have significant implications for the NHS.

References

Alderwick H, Dunn P, McKenna H, Walsh N and Ham C. (2016) *Sustainability and Transformation Plans in the NHS: How Are They Being Developed in Practice?* London: The King's Fund.

Allen P. (1995) Contracts in the NHS internal market. *Modern Law Review* 58: 321–342.

Allen P. (2002a) Plus ca change, plus c'est la meme chose: to the internal market and back in the British National Health Service. *Applied Health Economics and Health Policy* 1: 171–178.

Allen P. (2002b) A socio-legal and economic analysis of contracting in the NHS internal market using a case study of contracting for district nursing. *Social Science & Medicine* 54: 255–266.

Allen P. (2006) New localism in the English NHS: what is it for? *Health Policy* 79: 244–252.

Allen P. (2009a) Payment by results in the English NHS: the continuing challenges. *Public Money and Management* 29: 161–166.

Allen P. (2009b) Restructuring the NHS again: supply side reform in recent English healthcare policy. *Financial Accountability and Management* 25: 343–389.

Allen P. (2013) An economic analysis of the limits of market based reforms in the English NHS. *BMC Health Services Research* 13 Suppl 1: S1.

Allen P, Hughes D, Vincent-Jones P, Petsoulas C, Doheny S and Roberts J. (2016) Public contracts as accountability mechanisms: assuring quality in public health care in England and Wales. *Public Management Review* 18: 20–39.

Allen P and Jones L. (2011) Increasing the diversity of health care providers. In: Mays N, Dixon A and Jones L (eds) *Understanding New Labour's Market Reforms.* London: The King's Fund.

Allen P, Keen J, Wright JSF, Dempster P, Townsend J, Hutchings A, Street A and Verzulli R. (2012) Investigating the governance of acute hospitals in England: multi-site case study of NHS Foundation Trusts. *Journal of Health Services Research and Policy* 17: 94–100.

Allen P, Osipovic D, Shepherd E, Coleman A and Perkins N. (2014a) *Commissioning through Competition and Cooperation.* Interim Report. London: PRUComm.

Allen P, Osipovic D, Shepherd E, Coleman A, Perkins N and Garnett, E. (2016) *Commissioning through Competition and Cooperation.* Final Report. London: PRUComm.

Allen P, Osipovic D, Shepherd E, Coleman A, Perkins N, Garnett E and Williams L. (2017) Commissioning through competition and cooperation in the English NHS under the Health and Social Care Act 2012: evidence from a qualitative study of four Clinical Commissioning Groups. *BMJ Open* 7.

Allen P, Petsoulas C and Ritchie B. (2014b) *Study of the Use of Contractual Mechanisms in Commissioning.* Final Report. London PRUComm.

Arrow K. (1963) Uncertainty and the welfare economics of medical care. *American Economic Review* 53: 941–973.

Ashton T. (1998) Contracting for health services in New Zealand: a transaction cost analysis. *Social Science and Medicine* 46: 357–367.

Association of Directors of Public Health. (2015) English public health system 2015 survey – summary results. ADPH survey February 2015. www.adph.org.uk/wp-content/uploads/2015/06/ADPH-survey-summary-report-2015.pdf

Audit Commission. (2000) *The PCG Agenda: Early Progress of Primary Care Groups in 'The New NHS'.* London: Audit Commission.

Barr B, Higgerson J and Whitehead M. (2017) Investigating the impact of the English health inequalities strategy: time trend analysis. *British Medical Journal* 358: j3310.

Bartlett W and Le Grand J. (1993) The theory of quasi-markets. In: Le Grand J and Bartlett W (eds) *Quasi-Markets and Social Policy.* London: Macmillan.

Bate A, Donaldson C and Murtagh MJ. (2007) Managing to manage healthcare resources in the English NHS? What can health economics teach? What can health economics learn? *Health Policy* 84: 249–261.

Baum F. (2008) *The New Public Health.* Australia: Oxford University Press.

Bengtsson M and Kock S (2000) 'Coopetition' in business networks – to cooperate and compete simultaneously. *Industrial Marketing Management* 29: 411–426.

Benjamin P, Fung Lam W, Ostrom E and Shivakoti, G (1994) *Institutions, Incentives and Irrigation in Nepal. Decentralization: Finance and Management Project Report.* Burlington, VT: Associates in Rural Development.

Bennett M. (2015) *Commissioning in Local Government.* A research project for Local Partnerships: Local Partnerships (LGA and HM Treasury). http://localpartnerships.org.uk/wp-content/uploads/2016/05/Commissioning-in-local-government-BD.pdf

Berridge V, Gorsky M and Mold A. (2011) *Public Health in History,* Milton Keynes: Open University Press.

Best A, Greenhalgh T, Lewis S, Saul JE, Carroll S and Bitz J. (2012) Large-system transformation in health care: a realist review. *Milbank Q* 90: 421–456.

Best A and Holmes B. (2010) Systems thinking, knowledge and action: towards better models and methods. *Evidence & Policy: A Journal of Research, Debate and Practice* 6: 145–159.

Bevan G, Wyke S, Mays N, Abbot S, Goodwin N, Kilorran A, Malbon G, McLeod H, Posnett J and Raftery J. (1999) *Developing Primary Care in the New NHS: Lessons from Total Purchasing*. London: The King's Fund.

Bovens M. (2007) Analysing and assessing accountability: a conceptual framework. *European Law Journal* 13: 447–468.

Bradlow J and Coulter A. (1993) Effect of fundholding and indicative prescribing schemes on general practitioners' prescribing costs. *British Medical Journal* 307: 1186–1189.

Brandenburger A and Nalebuff B. (1996) *Co-opetition*. New York: Doubleday Dell Publishing Group.

Bravo Vergel Y and Ferguson B. (2006) Difficult commissioning choices: lessons from English primary care trusts. *Journal of Health Services Research and Policy* 11: 150–154.

Brennan S. (2019) The integrator: can councils be true partners in ICS? *Health Service Journal,* 21 February 2019.

British Medical Association. (1997) *Medical Involvement in the Commissioning Process: A Report of a National Study of Health Authorities and LMCs in England*. London: BMA.

British Medical Association. (2017) Funding for ill-health prevention and public health in the UK. www.bma.org.uk

Buck D. (2018) Local government spending on public health: death by a thousand cuts. London: The King's Fund. www.kingsfund.org.uk/blog

Byng R, Quinn C, Sheaff R, Samele C, Duggan S, Harrison D, Owens C, Smithson P, Wright C, Annison, J, Brown C, Taylor R, Henley W, Qureshi A, Shenton D, Porter I, Warrington C and Campbell J. (2012) COCOA: Care for Offenders, Continuity of Access Final Report. NIHR Service Delivery and Organisation programme.

Campbell F. (2010) The social determinants of health and the role of local government. Improvement and Development Agency. www.idea.gov.uk

Carding N. (2017) Previously blocked trust merger could be complete in a year. *Health Services Journal,* 27 September 2017.

Checkland K, Coleman A, Harrison S and Hiroch U. (2008). Practice-based Commissioning in the National Health Service: interim report of a qualitative study. University of Manchester, National Primary Care Research and Development Centre.

Checkland K, Coleman A, Harrison S and Hiroeh U. (2009) 'We can't get anything done because…': making sense of 'barriers' to practice-based commissioning. *Journal of Health Services Research and Policy* 14: 20–26.

Checkland K, Coleman A and Harrison S. (2011) When is a saving not a saving? The micro-politics of budgets and savings under practice-based commissioning. *Public Money and Management* 31: 241–248.

Checkland K, Coleman A, Segar J, McDermott I, Miller R, Wallace A, Petsoulas C, Peckham S and Harrison S. (2012) *Exploring the Early Workings of Emerging Clinical Commissioning Groups: Final Report.* London: PRUComm.

Checkland K, Allen P, Coleman A, Segar J, McDermott I, Harrison S, Petsoulas C and Peckham S. (2013a) Accountable to whom, for what? An exploration of the early development of Clinical Commissioning Groups in the English NHS. *BMJ Open* 3.

Checkland K, Coleman A, McDermott I, Segar J, Miller R, Petsoulas C, Wallace A, Harrison S and Peckham S. (2013b) Primary care-led commissioning: applying lessons from the past to the early development of Clinical Commissioning Groups in England. *British Journal of General Practice: Journal of the Royal College of General Practitioners* 63: e611–e619.

Checkland K, McDermott I, Coleman A and Perkins N. (2016) Complexity in the new NHS: longitudinal case studies of CCGs in England. *BMJ Open* 6.

Checkland K, Dam R, Hammond J, Coleman A, Segar J, Mays N and Allen P. (2017) Being autonomous and having space in which to act: commissioning in the 'New NHS' in England. *Journal of Social Policy* 47: 377–395.

Checkland K, Hammond J, Sutton M, Coleman A, Allen P, Mays N, Mason T, Wilding A, Warwick-Giles L and Hall A. (2018a) *Understanding the New Commissioning System in England: Contexts, Mechanisms and Outcomes. Final Report.* University of Manchester and London School of Hygiene and Tropical Medicine.

Checkland K, McDermott I, Coleman A, Warwick-Giles L, Bramwell D, Allen P and Peckham S. (2018b) Planning and managing primary care services: lessons from the NHS in England. *Public Money & Management* 38: 261–270.

Checkland K, Sutton M, Segar J, Allen P, Coleman A, Mays N, Hammond J, Mason T and Hall A. (2018c) *Understanding the New Commissioning System*. Manchester: University of Manchester.

Coase R. (1937) The nature of the firm. *Economica* 4: 386–405.

Coleman A, Checkland K, Harrison S and Dowswell G. (2009) *Practice-based Commissioning: Theory, Implementation and Outcome*. Final Report. University of Manchester: National Primary Care Research and Development Centre.

Coleman A, Checkland K, Harrison S and Hiroeh, U. (2010) Local histories and local sensemaking: a case of policy implementation in the English National Health Service. *Policy & Politics* 38: 289–306.

Coleman A, Checkland K, McDermott I and Harrison S. (2013) The limits of market-based reforms in the NHS: the case of alternative providers in primary care. *BMC Health Services Research* 13 Suppl 1: S3–S3.

Coleman A, Checkland K, Segar J, McDermott I, Harrison S and Peckham S. (2014) Joining it up? Health and Wellbeing Boards in English local governance: evidence from Clinical Commissioning Groups and Shadow Health and Wellbeing Boards. *Local Government Studies* 40: 560–580.

Coleman A, Dhesi S and Peckham S. (2016) Health and Well-Being Boards: the new system stewards. In: Exworthy M, Mannion R and Powell M (eds) *Dismantling the NHS? Evaluating the Impact of Health Reforms*. Bristol: Policy Press.

Competition Commission. (2013) *Decision on the Merger of the Royal Bournemouth and Christchurch Hospitals NHS Foundation Trust and Poole Hospital NHS Foundation Trust*. London: Competition Commission.

Corney RH and Kerrison S. (1997) Fundholding in the south Thames region. *British Journal of General Practice* 47: 553–556.

Courpasson D. (2000) Managerial strategies of domination: power in soft bureaucracies. *Organization Studies* 21: 141–161.

Cowton CJ and Drake JE. (1999a) Taking the lead in fundholding. *Journal of Management in Medicine* 13: 218–233.

Cowton CJ and Drake JE. (1999b) Went fundholding, going commissioning? Some evidence-based reflections on the prospects for primary care groups. *Public Money & Management* 19: 33–37.

Craig N, McGregor S, Drummond N, Fischbacher M and Iliffe S. (2002) Factors affecting the shift towards a 'primary care-led' NHS: a qualitative study. National Health Service. *British Journal of General Practice* 52: 895–900.

Crown Commercial Service. (2016) *The Public Contracts Regulations 2015. Guidance on the new light touch regime for health, social, education and certain other service contracts.* https://assets.publishing.service.gov.uk/government/uploads/system/uploads/attachment_data/file/560272/Guidance_on_Light_Touch_Regime_-_Oct_16.pdf

Croxson B. (1999) *Organisational Costs in the New NHS: An Introduction to the Transaction Costs and Internal Costs of Delivering Health Care.* London: Office of Health Economics.

Croxson B, Propper C and Perkins A. (2001) Do doctors respond to financial incentives? UK family doctors and the GP fundholder scheme. *Journal of Public Economics* 79: 375–398.

Curry N and Thorlby R. (2007) *Practice-Based Commissioning.* London: The King's Fund.

Daly M and Westwood S. (2017) Asset-based approaches, older people and social care: an analysis and critique. *Ageing and Society* 38: 1087–1099.

Davies A. (2004) Foundation Hospitals: a new approach to accountability and autonomy in the delivery of public services *Public Law:* 808–828.

Davies ACL. (2013) This time, it's for real: the Health and Social Care Act 2012. *The Modern Law Review* 76: 564–588.

Den Exter AP and Guy M. (2014) Market competition in health care markets in the Netherlands: some lessons for England? *Medical Law Review* 22: 255–273.

Department of Health. (1989) *Working for Patients.* White Paper. Cm 555 London: HMSO.

Department of Health. (2000) *The NHS Plan: A Plan for Investment, A Plan for Reform.* London: The Stationery Office.

Department of Health. (2003) Sustaining Innovation through New Personal Medical Services (PMS) Arrangements.

Department of Health. (2005) Department of Health website dh.gov.uk. London: Department of Health.

Department of Health. (2006a) *Health Reforms in England: Update and Commissioning Framework.* London: Department of Health.

Department of Health. (2006b) *Our Health, Our Care, Our Say: A New Direction for Community Services.* Cm 6737. London: The Stationery Office.

Department of Health. (2007a) *Brief for Health Reform Evaluation Programme.* London: Department of Health.

Department of Health. (2007b) *Options for the Future of Payment by Results 2008/9 to 2010/11.* London: Department of Health.

Department of Health. (2008) *Using the Commissioning for Quality and Innovation (CQUIN) Payment Framework.* London: Department of Health.

Department of Health. (2009) *The NHS in England: Operating Framework 2010–2011*. London: Department of Health.

Department of Health. (2010a) *Equity and Excellence: Liberating the NHS*. London: The Stationery Office.

Department of Health. (2010b) *Healthy Lives, Healthy People: Our Strategy for Public Health in England*. London: Department of Health.

Department of Health. (2010c) *Principles and Rules for Cooperation and Competition* (revised edition). London: Department of Health.

Department of Health (2011a). *Developing Clinical Commissioning Groups. Towards authorization*. London: Department of Health. https://assets.publishing.service.gov.uk/government/uploads/system/uploads/attachment_data/file/213725/dh_130318.pdf

Department of Health. (2011b) *Local Government's New Public Health Functions*. London: Department of Health.

Department of Health (2011c) *The New Public Health System: Summary*. https://assets.publishing.service.gov.uk/government/uploads/system/uploads/attachment_data/file/216715/dh_131897.pdf

Department of Health. (2012a) The Health and Social Care Act 2012 – An Overview. Factsheet A1, updated 30 April 2012. www.gov.uk/government/uploads/system/uploads/attachment_data/file/138257/A1.-Factsheet-Overview-240412.pdf

Department of Health. (2012b) New Focus for Public Health – the Health and Social Care Act 2012. Factsheet B4. London: Department of Health.

Department of Health. (2013a) *Developing a Specification for Lifestyle Weight Management Services: Best Practice Guidance for Tier 2 Services*. London: Department of Health.

Department of Health. (2013b) *Statutory Guidance on Joint Strategic Needs Assessments and Joint Health and Wellbeing Strategies*. London: Department of Health. https://assets.publishing.service.gov.uk/government/uploads/system/uploads/attachment_data/file/223842/Statutory-Guidance-on-Joint-Strategic-Needs-Assessments-and-Joint-Health-and-Wellbeing-Strategies-March-2013.pdf

Department of Health. (2014) Letter from Jane Ellison, Department of Health to Duncan Selbie and Professor David Heymann, Public Health England. 11 June 2014. https://assets.publishing.service.gov.uk/government/uploads/system/uploads/attachment_data/file/319708/PHE_remit_letter_pdf.pdf

Department of Health. (2015) Local Authority Public Health Grant Allocations 2015/16: Government Response to Public Consultation on In-Year Savings and Equality and Health Inequality Analysis. November 2015. London: Department of Health.

Department of Health. (2016) The Public Contracts Regulations 2015 and NHS Commissioners. www.gov.uk/government/uploads/system/uploads/attachment_data/file/561778/PCR_2015_and_NHS_commissioners_A.pdf

Dixon J, Goodwin N and Mays N. (1998) Accountability and total purchasing pilots. London: The King's Fund.

Dodge I and Doyle A. (2015) Letter to CCG Accountable Officers and CCG Clinical Chair: Delegated commissioning of primary medical services (Gateway ref. 04160).

Dowling B. (1997) Effect of fundholding on waiting times: database study. *British Medical Journal* 315: 290–292.

Drummond N, Iliffe S, McGregor S, Craig N and Fischbacher M. (2001) Can primary care be both patient-centred and community-led? *Journal of Management in Medicine* 15: 364–375.

Dunhill L. (2016) Stevens fires broadside against 'institutional self-interest'. *Health Services Journal*, 7 January 2016.

Durose C, Greasley S and Richardson L. (2009) *Changing Local Governance, Changing Citizens.* Bristol: Policy Press.

Dusheiko M, Gravelle H, Jacobs R and Smith PC. (2006) The effect of budgets on doctor behaviour: evidence from a natural experiment. *Journal of Health Economics* 25: 449–478.

Ennew C, Whynes D, Jolleys J and Robinson P. (1998) Entrepreneurship and innovation among GP fundholders. *Public Money & Management* 18: 59–64.

Enthoven A. (1985) Reflections on the management of the National Health Service. The Nuffield Provincial Hospitals Trust.

Erens B, Wistow G, Mounier-Jacl S, Douglas N, Jones L, Mannacorda T and Mays N. (2016) *Early Evaluation of the Integrated Care and Support Pioneers Programme.* Final Report. London: Policy Innovation Research Unit (PIRU).

Exworthy M, Frosini F, Jones L, Peckham S, Powell M, Greener I, Anand P and Holloway J. (2010) *Decentralisation and Performance: Autonomy and Incentives in Local Health Economies.* Technical Report. Southampton: NCCSDO.

Figueras J, Robinson R and Jakubowski E. (2005a) *Purchasing to Improve Health Systems Performance.* Maidenhead: Open University Press.

Figueras J, Robinson R and Jakubowski E. (2005b) Purchasing to improve health systems performance. *European Observatory on Health Systems and Policies.* Maidenhead: Open University Press.

Flynn R, Williams G and Pickard S. (1996) *Markets and Networks: Contracting in Community Health Services.* Buckingham: Open University Press.

Forder J, Knapp M, Hardy B, Kendall J, Matosevic T and Ware G. (2004) Prices, contracts and motivations: institutional arrangements in domiciliary care. *Policy & Politics* 32: 207–222.

France G, Taroni F and Donatini A. (2005) The Italian health-care system. *Health Economics* 14: S187–S202.

Fulop N, Mowlem A and Edwards N. (2005) *Building Integrated Care: Lessons from the UK and Elsewhere.* London: The NHS Confederation.

Gadsby EW, Peckham S, Coleman A, Bramwell D, Perkins N and Jenkins LM. (2017a) Commissioning for health improvement following the 2012 health and social care reforms in England: what has changed? *BMC Public Health* 17: 211.

Gadsby EW, Peckham S, Coleman A, Bramwell D, Perkins N and Jenkins LM. (2017b) Commissioning for health improvement following the 2012 health and social care reforms in England: what has changed? *BMC Public Health* 17: 211.

Gadsby EW, Peckham S, Coleman A, Segar J, Perkins N, Jenkins L and Bramwell D. (2014) PHOENIX: Public Health and Obesity in England – the New Infrastructure Examined. First Interim Report: The Scoping Review. Policy Research Unit in Commissioning and the Healthcare System.

Gains F, Greasley S and Stoker G. (2004) Local political management. *New Economy* 11: 84–89.

Gibson C, McKean M and Ostrom E. (2000) *People and Forests: Communities, Institutions and Governance.* Cambridge, MA: MIT Press.

Gibson J, Sutton M, Spooner S and Checkland K. (2017) *Ninth National GP Worklife Survey.* London: Policy Research Unit in Commissioning and the Healthcare System.

Glennerster H, Matsaganis M, Owens P and Hancock S. (1994a) GP fundholding: wild card or winning hand? In: Robinson R and Le Grand J (eds) *Evaluating the NHS Reforms.* Hermitage: Policy Journals, 74–107.

Glennerster H, Matsaganis M, Owens P and Hancock S. (1994b) *Implementing GP Fundholding: Wild Card or Winning Hand?* Buckingham: Open University Press.

Goddard M and Mannion R. (1998) From competition to co-operation: new economic relationships in the National Health Service. *Health Economics* 7: 105–119.

Goodwin N, Mays N, McLeod H, Malbon G and Raftery J. (1998) Evaluation of total purchasing pilots in England and Scotland and implications for primary care groups in England: personal interviews and analysis of routine data. *British Medical Journal* 317: 256–259.

Gorsky M, Lock K and Hogarth S. (2014) Public health and English local government: historical perspectives on the impact of 'returning home'. *Journal of Public Health* 36: 546–551.

Green MA, Dorling D, Minton J and Pickett KE. (2017) Could the rise in mortality rates since 2015 be explained by changes in the number of delayed discharges of NHS patients? *Journal of Epidemiology and Community Health*,71: 1068–1071.

Greener I and Powell M. (2009) The evolution of choice policies in UK housing, education and health policy. *Journal of Social Policy* 38: 63–81.

Griffiths S, Jewell T and Donnelly P. (2005) Public health in practice: the three domains of public health. *Public Health* 119: 907–913.

Gunn LA. (1978) Why is implementation so difficult? *Management Services in Government* 33: 169–176.

Ham C. (2017) *What are STPs and Why Do They Matter? Big Election Questions.* London: The King's Fund. www.kingsfund.org.uk/publications/articles/big-election-questions-stps

Ham C. (2018) *A Progress Report on Integrated Care Systems.* London: The King's Fund. www.kingsfund.org.uk/blog/2018/03/progress-report-integrated-care-systems

Hammond J, Hall A and Checkland K. (2017) *Understanding the New Commissioning System in England: Contexts, Mechanisms and Outcomes. Work Stream 2 – Tracer Short Report Sexual Health Services.* Manchester: University of Manchester.

Hazell W. (2014) Monitor: Role for competition in new provider landscape. *Health Services Journal,* November 2014.

Health and Social Care Act. (2012) *Chapter 7.* London: The Stationery Office.

Hiam L, Harrison D, McKee M and Dorling D. (2018) Why is life expectancy in England and Wales 'stalling'? *Journal of Epidemiology and Community Health.* 72: 404–408.

Hine CE and Bachmann MO. (1997) What does locality commissioning in Avon offer? Retrospective descriptive evaluation. *British Medical Journal* 314: 1246–1250.

Hirschman A. (1970) *Exit, Voice, and Loyalty: Responses to Decline in Firms, Organizations, and States.* Cambridge, MA: Harvard University Press.

Hodkinson P and Hodkinson H. (2001) The strengths and limitations of case study research. In: *Learning and Skills Development Agency Conference: Making an Impact on Policy and Practice.* Leeds: University of Leeds.

House of Commons Health and Social Care Committee. (2018) *Integrated Care: Organisations, Partnerships and Systems. Seventh Report of Session 2017–19.* London: House of Commons.

House of Commons Health Committee. (2014) *Public Health England – Eighth Report of Session 2013–14* (HC840). London: The Stationery Office Ltd.

House of Commons Health Committee. (2015) Public Health Post-2013 Inquiry Launch. UK Parliament.

House of Commons Health Committee. (2016) Public Health Post-2013. Second Report of Session 2016–17. www.parliament.uk/healthcom

Howie JG, Heaney DJ and Maxwell M. (1993) The chief scientist reports … evaluation of the Scottish shadow fund-holding project: first results. *Health Bulletin* 51: 94–105.

Hughes C. (2015) The rewards and challenges of setting up a Tier 3 adult weight management service in primary care. *British Journal of Obesity* 1: 1–40.

Hughes D and Dingwall R. (1990) Sir Henry Maine, Joseph Stalin and the reorganisation of the national health service. *Journal of Social Welfare Law* 12: 296–309.

Hughes D and Vincent-Jones P. (2008) Schisms in the church: NHS systems and institutional divergence in England and Wales. *Journal of Health and Social Behaviour* 49: 400–416.

Hughes D, McHale J and Griffiths L. (1997) Settling contract disputes in the National Health Service: formal and informal pathways. In: Flynn R and Williams G (eds) *Contracting for Health: Quasi-Markets and the National Health Service.* Oxford: Oxford University Press.

Hunter DJ, Perkins N, Visram S, Adams L, Finn R, Forrest A and Gosling, J. (2018) Evaluating the leadership role of Health and Wellbeing Boards as drivers of health improvement and integrated care across England. Final report. Stockton-on-Tees: Durham University.

Hupe PL and Hill MJ. (2015) 'And the rest is implementation': comparing approaches to what happens in policy processes beyond Great Expectations. *Public Policy and Administration* 31: 103–121.

Iacobucci G. (2014) Raiding the public health budget. *British Medical Journal* 348: 2274.

Iacobucci G. (2016) Public health – the frontline cuts begin. *British Medical Journal* 352–i272.

Iacobucci G. (2017) NHS in 2017: where next? *British Medical Journal* 356.:j331.

Illman J and Dunhill L. (2016) Stevens: give any extra funding to social care over NHS. *Health Service Journal,* 17 June 2016.

Institute of Medicine. (2002) *The Future of the Public's Health in the 21st Century.* Washington, DC: National Academies Press.

Jenkins LM, Bramwell D, Coleman A, Gadsby E W, Peckham S, Perkins N and Segar J. (2016) Integration, influence and change in public health: findings from a survey of Directors of Public Health in England. *Journal of Public Health* 38: e201–e208.

Joskow P. (1987) Contract duration and relationship-specific investments: empirical evidence from coal markets. *American Economic Review* 77: 168–185.

Kammerling RM and Kinnear A. (1996) The extent of the two tier service for fundholders. *British Medical Journal* 312: 1399–1401.

Kneale D, Rojas-Garcia A, Raine R and Thomas J. (2017) The use of evidence in English local public health decision-making: a systematic scoping review. *Implementation Science* 12, doi:10.1186/s13012-017-0577-9

Kodner DL and Spreeuwenberg C. (2002) Integrated care: meaning, logic, applications, and implications – a discussion paper. *International Journal of Integrated Care* 2: e12.

Krachler N and Greer I. (2015) When does marketisation lead to privatisation? Profit-making in English health services after the 2012 Health Care Act. *Social Science and Medicine* 124: 215–223.

Kurunmaki L. (1999) Professional vs. financial capital in the field of health care: struggles for the redistribution of power and control. *Accounting, Organisations and Society* 24: 95–124.

Lambert MF and Sowden S. (2016) Revisiting the risks associated with health and healthcare reform in England: perspective of Faculty of Public Health members. *Journal of Public Health* 38: e438–e445.

Langfield-Smith K. (2008) The relations between transactional characteristics, trust and risk in the start-up phase of a collaborative alliance. *Management Accounting Research* 19: 344–364.

Lapsley I, Llewellyn S and Grant J. (1997) GP Fundholders: Agents of Change. Edinburgh: The Institute of Chartered Accountants of Scotland.

Le Grand J and Bartlett W. (1993) *Quasi-Markets and Social Policy*. London: Macmillan.

Learmonth M. (1997) Managerialism and public attitudes towards UK NHS managers. *Journal of Management in Medicine* 11: 214–221.

Lewis J. (1997) *Independent Contractors: GPs and the GP Contract in the Post-War Period*. Manchester: University of Manchester.

Lintern S. (2017) Internal market and FT 'islands' hamper safe care, says Hunt. *Health Services Journal*, published online 28 November 2017.

Llewellyn S. (2001) 'Two-way windows': clinicians as medical managers. *Organization Studies* 22: 593–623.

Local Government Association. (2016) *Health in All Policies: A Manual for Local Government*. London: Local Government Association.

Local Government Association. (2018) Public health transformation five years on. Transformation in action. www.local.gov.uk/sites/default/files/documents/22.14%20Public%20health%205%20years%20on_Web.pdf

Longley D. (1990) Diagnostic dilemmas: accountability in the NHS. *Public Law*: 527–552.

Macaulay S. (1963) Non-contractual relations and busness: a preliminary study. *American Sociological Review* 28: 55–67.

Macneil I. (1981) Economic analysis of contractual relations: its shortfalls and the need for a rich classificatory apparatus. *Northwestern University Law Review* 75: 10–22.

Majeed A, Rawaf S and De Maeseneer J. (2012) Primary care in England: coping with financial austerity. *British Journal of General Practice: The Journal of the Royal College of General Practitioners* 62: 625–626.

Malbon G and Mays N. (1998) Total recall: what can total purchasing pilots teach PCGs? *British Journal of Health Care Management* 4: 428–430.

Mannion R. (2008) General practitioner commissioning in the English National Health Service: continuity, change, and future challenges. *International Journal of Health Services* 38: 717–730.

Marini G and Street A. (2007) A transaction costs analysis of changing contractual relations in the English NHS. *Health Policy* 83: 17–26.

Marks L, Cave S and Hunter DJ. (2010) Public health governance: views of key stakeholders. *Public Health* 124: 55–59.

Marks L, Cave S, Hunter D, Mason J, Peckham S and Wallace A. (2011) Governance for health and wellbeing in the English NHS. *Journal of Health Services Research & Policy* 16: 14–21.

Marks L, Hunter D, Scalabrini S, Gray J, McCafferty S, Payne N, Peckham S, Salway S and Thokala P. (2015) The return of public health to local government in England: changing the parameters of the public health prioritization debate? *Public Health* 129: 1194–1203.

Marmot M. (2010) *Fair Society, Healthy Lives: The Marmot Review*. Strategic Review of Health Inequalities in England post-2010. www.ucl.ac.uk/marmotreview

Masters R, Anwar E, Collins B, Cookson R and Capewell S. (2017) Return on investment of public health interventions: a systematic review. *Journal of Epidemiology and Community Health* 71: 827–834.

Mays N. (1996) *Total Purchasing: A Profile of National Pilot Projects*. London: The King's Fund.

Mays N, Goodwin N, Killoran A and Malbon, G. (1998a) *Total Purchasing: A Step Towards Primary Care Groups: National Evaluation of Total Purchasing Pilot Projects.* London: The King's Fund.

Mays N, Goodwin N and Mabon G. (1998b) *What Were the Achievements of Total Purchasing Pilots in Their First Year and How Can They Be Explained?* London: The King's Fund.

Mays N, Wyke S, Malbon G and Goodwin N. (2001) *The Purchasing of Health Care by Primary Care Organisations: An Evaluation and Guide to Future Policy.* Birmingham: Open University Press.

McCallum A, Brommels T, Robinson R, Bergman S-E and Palu T. (2006) The impact of primary care purchasing in Europe: a comparative case study of primary care reform. In: Saltman RB, Rica A and Boema W (eds) *Primary Care in the Driver's Seat? Organisational Reform in European Primary Care.* Maidenhead: Open University Press.

McDermott I, Coleman A, Perkins N, Osipovic D, Petsoulas C and Checkland K. (2015) *Exploring the GP 'Added Value' in Commissioning: What Works, in What Circumstances, and How?* Final Report. London: PRUComm.

McDermott I, Checkland K, Coleman A, Osipovič D, Petsoulas C and Perkins N. (2016a) Engaging GPs in commissioning: realist evaluation of the early experiences of Clinical Commissioning Groups in the English NHS. *Journal of Health Services Research & Policy* 22: 4–11.

McDermott I, Checkland K, Warwick-Giles L and Coleman A. (2016b) *Understanding Primary Care Co-commissioning: Uptake, Scope of Activity and Process of Change.* Interim Report. London: PRUComm.

McDermott I, Warwick-Giles L, Gore O, Moran V, Bramwell D, Coleman A and Checkland K. (2018) *Understanding Primary Care Co-Commissioning: Uptake, Development, and Impacts.* Final Report. London: PRUComm.

McHale J, Hughes D and Griffiths L. (1997) Conceptualising contractual disputes in the National Health Service internal market. In: Deakin S and Michie J (eds) *Contracts. Co-operation and Competition: Studies in Economics, Management and Law.* Oxford: Oxford University Press.

Miller R, Peckham S, Checkland K, Coleman A, McDermott I, Harrison S and Segar J. (2012) *Clinical Engagement in Primary Care-Led Commissioning: A Review of the Evidence.* London: Policy Research Unit in Commissioning and the Healthcare System (PRUComm).

Miller R, Peckham S, Checkland K, Coleman A, McDermott I and Harrison S. (2015) What happens when GPs engage in commissioning? Two decades of experience in the English NHS. *Journal of Health Services Research & Policy* online first, 21:126–33.

Mills & Reeve. (2016) *Commissioning Clinical Health Services: Most Capable Provider versus Light Touch Regime?* 25 January 2016, www.mills-reeve.com/commissioning-clinical-health-services-most-capable-provider-versus-light-touch-regime-01-25-2016/

Monitor. (2013a) *Local Price Setting and Contracting Practices for NHS Services without a Nationally Mandated Price.* London: Monitor.

Monitor. (2013b) *Local Price Setting and Contracting Practices for NHS Services without a Nationally Mandated Price: A Research Paper.* London: Monitor.

Monitor. (2014a) *Capitation: A Potential New Payment Model to Enable Integrated Care.* London: NHS England.

Monitor. (2014b) *Choice and Competition Licence Conditions: Guidance for Providers of NHS-Funded Services.* London: Monitor.

Monitor. (2015a) Complying with Monitor's integrated care requirements. www.gov.uk/government/publications/integrated-care-how-to-comply-with-monitors-requirements/complying-with-monitors-integrated-care-requirements

Monitor. (2015b) Integrated care licence condition: consultation on draft guidance for providers of NHS-funded services. Issued on 14 January 2015; Deadline for responses: 13 February 2015. London: Monitor.

Monitor. (2015c) *Multilateral Gain/Loss Sharing: A Financial Mechanism to Support Collaborative Service Reform.* London: NHS England.

Monitor and NHS England. (2014) 2015/16 Mental Health TED Workshop. https://assets.publishing.service.gov.uk/government/uploads/system/uploads/attachment_data/file/357578/Mental_Health_TED_Workshop.pdf

Moran V, Allen P, McDermott I, Checkland K, Warwick-Giles L, Gore O, Bramwell D and Coleman A. (2017a) How are Clinical Commissioning Groups managing conflicts of interest under primary care co-commissioning in England? A qualitative analysis. *BMJ Open* 7.

Moran V, Checkland K, Coleman A, Spooner S, Gibson J and Sutton M. (2017b) General practitioners' views of clinically led commissioning: cross-sectional survey in England. *BMJ Open* 7.

Munton T, Martin A, Marrero I, Llewellyn A, Gibson K and Gomersall A. (2011) *Getting out of Hospital? The Evidence for Shifting Acute Inpatient and Day Care Services from Hospitals into the Community.* London: The Health Foundation.

Newman M, Bangpan M, Kalra N, Mays N, Kwan I and Roberts A. (2012) *Commissioning in Health, Education and Social Care: Models, Research Bibliography and In-Depth Review of Joint Commissioning between Health and Social Care Agencies.* London: EPPI-Centre, Social Science.

NHS Commissioning Board. (2012a) Clinical Commissioning Groups HR Guide. NHS Commissioning Board.

NHS Commissioning Board. (2012b) Commissioning fact sheet for Clinical Commissioning Groups. NHS Commissioning Board.

NHS Commissioning Board. (2012c) Towards establishment: creating responsive and accountable Clinical Commissioning Groups. NHS Commissioning Board. www.england.nhs.uk/wp-content/uploads/2017/05/towards-establishment.pdf

NHS Commissioning Board. (2012d) Local area teams. Staff briefing pack 20 June 2012. NHS Commissioning Board. www.england.nhs.uk/wp-content/uploads/2012/06/lat-senates-pack.pdf

NHS Digital. (2018) *Data Dictionary: Strategic Health Authority.* Leeds: NHS Digital.

NHS England. (2014a) *Five Year Forward View.* London: NHS England.

NHS England. (2014b) *Managing Conflicts of Interest: Statutory Guidance for CCGs.* London: NHS England.

NHS England. (2014c) *Next Steps towards Primary Care Co-commissioning.* London: NHS England.

NHS England. (2015a) NHS Standard Contract Guidance to Template Alliance Agreement.

NHS England. (2015b) Primary care co-commissioning update webinar. 14 July 2015, https://www.england.nhs.uk/commissioning/wp-content/uploads/sites/12/2015/08/140715-pcc-com-webinar.pdf

NHS England. (2016a) *Managing Conflicts of Interest: Revised Statutory Guidance for CCGs.* Leeds: NHS England.

NHS England. (2016b) NHS Standard Contract Template Alliance Agreement for Virtual MCP/PACS models. https://www.england.nhs.uk/wp-content/uploads/2017/08/3b.-170802-Alliance-Agreement.pdf

NHS England. (2017a) Delegated commissioning case studies. www.england.nhs.uk/commissioning/pc-co-comms/dc-cs/

NHS England. (2017b) Managing Conflicts of Interest: Revised statutory guidance for CCGs 2017. Leeds: NHS England.

NHS England. (2017c) *Next Steps on the NHS Five Year Forward View.* London: NHS England.

NHS England. (2017d) Template Alliance Agreement for accountable models – overview.www.england.nhs.uk/wp-content/uploads/2017/08/1693_DraftMCP-3a_A.pdf

NHS England. (2018a) Commissioning. What is Commissioning? www.england.nhs.uk/commissioning/

NHS England. (2018b) Draft ICP Contract: A Consultation. NHS England Publications Gateway Reference: 07883.

NHS England. (2019) Contracting Arrangements for Integrated Care Providers – Response to Consultation. London: NHS England.

NHS England and NHS Improvement. (2016) *NHS Operational Planning and Contracting Guidance 2017–2019*. London: NHS England and NHS Improvement.

NHS England and NHS Improvement. (2018a) *Payment System Reform Proposals for 2019/20*. A joint publication by NHS England and NHS Improvement. London: NHS Improvement.

NHS England and NHS Improvement. (2018b) *Refreshing NHS Plans for 2018/19*. London: NHS England and NHS Improvement.

NHS England and NHS Improvement. (2019) *NHS Long Term Plan*. London: NHS England and NHS Improvement.

NHS England, NHS Improvement, Care Quality Commission, et al. (2015) Delivering the Forward View: NHS Planning Guidance 2016/17–2020/21. London.

NHS England. (2016) *Public Contracts Regulations 2015: For Information not Statement of Policy*. London: NHS England.

NHS Improvement. (2016) *Briefing for Clinical Commissioning Groups: Options for Selecting Providers and Awarding Contracts*. London: NHS Improvement.

NICE. (2014) *Obesity: Identification, Assessment and Management*. Guidelines CG189. London: NICE.

Nicholson D. (2010) *Letter to all Chief Executives and Arm's Length Bodies: Equity and Excellence: Liberating the NHS – Managing the Transition*. London: Department of Health.

Osborne SP and Radnor Z. (2016) The New Public Governance and innovation in public services. In: Torfing J (ed) *Enhancing Public Innovation by Transforming Public Governance*. Cambridge: Cambridge University Press 54–70.

Osipovic D, Allen P, Shepherd E, Coleman A, Perkins N, Williams L, Sanderson M and Checkland K. (2016) Interrogating Institutional Change: Actors' Attitudes to Competition and Cooperation in Commissioning Health Services in England. *Public Administration* 94: 823–838.

Osipovic D, Allen P, Petsoulas C and Moran V. (2017) *Next Steps in Commissioning through Competition and Cooperation (2016–2017)*. Additional Report. London: PRUComm.

Osipovic D, Allen P, Sanderson M, Moran V and Checkland K. (2019) The regulation of competition and procurement in the National Health Service 2015–2018: enduring hierarchical control and the limits of juridification. *Health Economics, Policy and Law*, doi: 10.1017/S1744133119000240. Published online by Cambridge University Press: 29 October 2019, https://doi.org/10.1017/S1744133119000264

Ostrom E. (2005) *Understanding Institutional Diversity*. Princeton, NJ: Princeton University Press.

Ostrom E. (2010) Beyond markets and states: polycentric governance of complex economic systems. In: Grandin K (ed) *Les Prix Nobel: The Nobel Prizes 2009*. Stockholm: Nobel Foundation.

Palmer N and Mills A. (2005) Contracts in the real world: case studies from Southern Africa. *Soc Sci Med Social Science and Medicine* 60: 2505–2514.

Parkhurst JO and Abeysinghe S. (2016) What constitutes 'good' evidence for public health and social policy-making? From hierarchies to appropriateness. *Social Epistemology* 30: 665–679.

Pawson R. (2013) *The Science of Evaluation: A Realist Manifesto*. London: Sage.

Peckham S and Exworthy M. (2003) *Primary Care in the UK: Policy, Organisation, and Management*. Hampshire, UK:Palgrave Macmillan.

Peckham S, Gadsby E, Coleman A, Jenkins L, Perkins N, Rutter H, Segar J and Bramwell D. (2015) *PHOENIX: Public Health and Obesity in England – the New Infrastructure Examined*. Second Interim Report. London: PRUComm.

Peckham S, Gadsby EW, Coleman A, Jenkins L, Perkins N, Bramwell D, Ogilvie J Rutter H and Segar J. (2016) PHOENIX: Public Health and Obesity in England – the New Infrastructure Examined. Final Report. Policy Research Unit on Commissioning and the Healthcare System. http://blogs.lshtm.ac.uk/prucomm/files/2016/07/PHOENIX-report-final.pdf

Petsoulas C, Allen P, Hughes D, Vincent-Jones P and Roberts J. (2011) The use of standard contracts in the English National Health Service: a case study analysis. *Social Science & Medicine* 73:. 185–92.

Petsoulas C, Allen P, Checkland K, Coleman A, Segar J, Peckham S and McDermott I. (2014) Views of NHS commissioners on commissioning support provision: evidence from a qualitative study examining the early development of Clinical Commissioning Groups in England. *BMJ Open* 4: e005970.

Place M, Posnett J and Street A. (1998) The transaction costs of total purchasing pilots. London: The King's Fund.

Plsek PE and Greenhalgh T. (2001) The challenge of complexity in health care. *British Medical Journal* 323: 625–8.

Posnett J, Goodwin N, Griffiths J, Killoran A, Malbon G, Mays N, Place M and Street A. (1998) The transaction costs of total purchasing. National Evaluation of Total Purchasing Pilot Project Working Paper. London.

Pressman JL and Wildavsky AB. (1973) *Implementation: How Great Expectations in Washington are Dashed in Oakland.* Berkeley: University of California Press.

Propper C, Croxson B and Shearer A. (2002) Waiting times for hospital admissions: the impact of GP fundholding. *Journal of Health Economics* 21: 227–252.

Public Health England. (2015) *National Mapping of Weight Management Services: Provision of Tier 2 and Tier 3 Services in England.* London: PHE.

Public Health England. (2018) Sexually transmitted infections and screening for chlamydia in England, 2017. *Health Protection Report* Vol 12, No 20, 8 June 2018. London: PHE.

Raftery J, Robinson R, Mulligan JA and Forrest S. (1996) Contracting in the NHS quasi-market. *Health Economics* 5: 353–362.

RAND Europe and Ernst and Young. (2012) *National Evaluation of the Department of Health's Integrated Care Pilots.* Cambridge: RAND Europe.

Redfern J and Bowling A. (2000) Efficiency of care at the primary–secondary interface: variations with GP fundholding. *Health Place* 6: 15–23.

Regen E, Smith J, Goodwin N, McLeod H and Shapiro J. (2001) Passing on the baton: final report of a national evaluation of primary care groups and trusts. University of Birmingham, Health Services Management Centre.

Rhodes RAW. (2007) Understanding governance: ten years on. *Organization Studies* 28: 1243–1264.

Riches N, Coleman A, Gadsby EW and Peckham S. (2015) *The Role of Local Authorities in Health Issues: A Policy Document Analysis.* London: PRUComm, Policy Research Unit on Commissioning and the Healthcare System.

Roberts J. (1993) Managing markets. *Journal of Public Health* 14: 305–310.

Robertson R, Holder H, Bennett L, Curry N, Ross S and Naylor C. (2015) *Primary Care Co-commissioning.* London: The King's Fund.

Robertson R, Holder H, Ross S, Naylor C and Machaqueiro S. (2016) *Clinical Commissioning GPs in Charge?* London: The King's Fund and the Nuffield Trust.

Royal College of General Practitioners and NHS Clinical Commissioners. (2014) The risks and opportunities for CCGs when co-commissioning primary care: things to consider when making your decision. 1–13. www.nhscc.org/wp-content/uploads/2014/12/FINAL-NHSCC_RCGP-Risks-and-opportunities-for-CCGs-in-primary-care-commissioning-1.121.pdf

Ruane S. (2014) Democratic engagement in the local NHS. London, Democratic Audit UK; Centre for Health and the Public Interest. www.democraticaudit.com

Rutten F. (2004) The impact of healthcare reform in the Netherlands. *PharmacoEconomics* 22: 65–71.

Rutter H, Savona N, Glonti K, Bibby J, Cummins S, Finegood DT, Greaves F, Harper L, Hawe P, Moore L, Petticrew M, Rehfuess E, Shiell A, Thomas J and White M. (2017) The need for a complex systems model of evidence for public health. *The Lancet* 390: 2602–2604.

Sabel C. (1991) Studied trust. In: Pyke F (ed) *Industrial Districts and Local Economic Regeneration.* Geneva:International Institute of Labour Studies.

Sanderson M, Allen P and Osipovic D. (2017) The regulation of competition in the National Health Service (NHS): what difference has the Health and Social Care Act 2012 made? *Health Economics Policy and Law* 12: 1–19.

Skelcher C and Torfing J. (2000) Improving democratic governance through institutional design: civic participation and democratic ownership in Europe *Regulation and Governance* 4: 71–91.

Smith A. (1776) *An Inquiry into the Nature and Causes of the Wealth of Nations.* London: Methuen.

Smith J, Curry N, Mays N and Dixon, J. (2010) *Where Next for Commissioning in the English NHS?* London: The King's Fund and the Nuffield Trust.

Smith J and Mays N. (2007) Primary care organizations in New Zealand and England: tipping the balance of the health system in favour of primary care? *International Journal of Health Planning and Management* 22: 3–19.

Smith J, Regen E, Shapiro J and Baines D. (2000) National evaluation of general practitioner commissioning pilots: lessons for primary care groups. *British Journal of General Practice* 50: 469–472.

Smith J, Mays N, Dixon J, Goodwin N, Lewis R, McClelland S, McLeod H and Wyke S. (2004) *A Review of the Effectiveness of Primary Care-Led Commissioning and Its Place in the NHS*. London: The Health Foundation.

Stewart J and Ranson S. (1988) Management in the public domain. *Public Money & Management* 8: 13–19.

Stokes J, Kristensen SR, Checkland K and Bower P. (2016) Effectiveness of multidisciplinary team case management: difference-in-differences analysis. *BMJ Open* 6.

Stopforth S. (2014) Healthy Dialogues round table write-up. New Local Government Network, London. www.nlgn.org.uk/public/wp-content/uploads/150115-Healthy-Dialogues_Roundtable-Write-Up1.pdf

Storey J, Holti R, Hartley J, Marshall M and Matharu T. (2018) Clinical leadership in service redesign using Clinical Commissioning Groups: a mixed-methods study. *NIHR Health Services and Delivery Research*. www.journalslibrary.nihr.ac.uk/hsdr/hsdr06020#/abstract

Sullivan H. (2007) Interpreting 'community leadership' in English local government. *Policy & Politics* 35: 141–161.

Surender R and Fitzpatrick R. (1999) Will doctors manage? Lessons from general practice fundholding. *Policy & Politics* 27: 491–502.

Sussex J and Street A. (2004) *Activity-Based Financing for Hospitals: English Policy and International Experience*. London: Office of Health Economics.

The Centre for Local Economic Strategies. (2014) *Austerity Uncovered: Final Report*, prepared by the Centre for Local Economic Strategies, Presented to TUC. December 2014. https://cles.org.uk/wp-content/uploads/2016/10/TUC-Final-Report.pdf

The Health Foundation. (2018) *X Factor for Evidence for the Public's Health: Exploring Why We Need to Use Different Kinds of Evidence to Improve the Public's Health*. London: The Health Foundation.

Thomas R and West D. (2017) STPs will end the purchaser–provider split, says Stevens. *Health Services Journal*. February 2017.

Tuohy C. (1999) *Accidental Logics: The Dynamics of Change in the Health Care Arena in the United States, Britain and Canada*. Oxford: Oxford University Press.

Vincent-Jones P. (2006) *The New Public Contracting*. Oxford: Oxford University Press.

Walker J and Mathers N. (2002) The impact of a general practice group intervention on prescribing costs and patterns. *British Journal of General Practice* 52: 181–186.

Watkins J, Wulaningsih W, Da Zhou C, Marshall D C, Sylianteng G D C, Dela Rosa PG, Miguel VA, Raine R, King LP and Maruthappu M. (2017) Effects of health and social care spending constraints on mortality in England: a time trend analysis. *BMJ Open* 7.

Weick KE. (1979) *The Social Psychology of Organizing.* Reading, MA: Addison-Wesley Publishing Company.

Weiss CH. (1997) Theory-based evaluation: past, present, and future. *New Directions for Evaluation* 1997: 41–55.

Weiss CH. (1998) *Evaluation.* Upper Saddle River, NJ: Prentice-Hall.

West D. and Calkin, S. (2014). Revealed: NHS England's new area team structure, *Health Service Journal*, 1 October 2014.

Wilkin D, Gillam S and Smith K. (2001) Primary care groups: tackling organisational change in the new NHS. *British Medical Journal* 322: 1464–1467.

Williamson OE. (1975) *Markets and Hierarchies: Analysis and Antitrust Implications.* New York: Free Press.

Williamson OE. (1985) *The Economic Institutions of Capitalism.* New York: Free Press.

Wilson RPH, Hatcher J, Barton S and Walley, T. (1999) The association of some practice characteristics with antibiotic prescribing. *Pharmacoepidemiology & Drug Safety* 8: 15–21.

Wyke S, Hewison J, Elton R, Posnett J, Macleod L and Ross-McGill H. (2001) Does general practitioner involvement in commissioning maternity care make a difference? *Journal of Health Services Research and Policy* 6: 99–104.

Yin RK. (2009) *Case Study Research: Design and Methods.* Los Angeles: Sage Publications.

Index